OVEREATING UNPLUGGED

It *ain't* just the food

Jill Bonney

www.overeatingunplugged.com

Mention of specific companies or organizations in this book does not imply endorsement, nor does their mention imply their endorsement of this book.

This publication contains the opinions and ideas of its author. It is sold on the basis that the reader should consult his or her medical, health, or other competent professional before drawing inference from or acting upon ideas and suggestions in this book. The author does not accept any legal responsibility for any personal injury, damage or loss from use or misuse of information in this book. Anyone making a change in their diet should consult their GP especially if pregnant, infirm, elderly or under 16.

www.overeatingunplugged.com

Originally published as Diet Detective.

Dedications

For the many people who have trod the path to my door, my wonderful clients, you have each and every one of you moved me deeply with your spirit of continual perseverance, whether you have succeeded or struggle still. Working with people is a two way process: as much as is given, is received, and I am grateful beyond measure for the privilege of your trust and numerous heart filled connections.

For my Mum and Dad, who are definitely different, and gave me my own slightly crazy angle on things.

And for Dawn who lost fifteen stone and changed her life to keep it that way.

Overeating Unplugged

It *ain't* just the food!

Names and places have been changed throughout to preserve confidentiality and avoid identification.

FORWARD!

What often gets overlooked is that the process of losing weight and getting slim is separate from the process of maintenance and weight holding. It's not just the diet or eating regime that needs changing but aspects of the lifestyle and mindset that keep that change in place. Plus you have to want whatever being slimmer and healthier gives you, and does for you, one percent more than the extra helping in front of you, enough of the time, over time. Sustained motivation... is usually the sticking point. If this wasn't the case, for most of us it would have been a wrap after the first diet. Job done.

Somehow though, however much we want the results, something doesn't quite work or the willpower we might draw on in other areas of our lives seems to let us down at some point or other: either then we do not want slimness and all the great things that go with it as much as we believed, or there are unseen tripwires along the way. Each of us has our own array of eating behaviours, and what we'll be tracking throughout is the minefield of scenarios that waylay our best intentions, time and again. Once you know the terrain, you will be far better equipped to sidestep the pitfalls and navigate your way through to lasting success. A lot of this involves plain common sense, but getting a handle on what's really been going on and putting it altogether will spark more than a few lightbulb moments to take you through. It will be a process of enlightenment, as well as getting lighter. And as you become your own best eating behaviour detective, the feel good factor will take you far further than willpower.

The extra good news is that the effort and focus we use to get there and stay there ripples into every area of our lives. We achieve singularity of purpose and strength of mind. We become as good as our word, can rely on ourselves, and so become personally accountable. This creates a peace of mind, and an inner stillness. This stillness is our ultimate healing. It is the Holy Grail of nourishment, and once we have it in our grasp, the temporary emotional stop gap that overeating provides, gets seen for what it is... a temporary stop gap.

It's not just about getting lighter, or looking better, feeling better, several sizes down the clothes scale. It's not just a physical process but a literal, mental, emotional and all systems launching transformation which will be the best investment you ever made.

What's it all about?

For the most part, *what* you eat is pivotal to the plot. But the issue of how we manage to eat more than we need equally begs the question of *when, where, who with* and *why?*

A lot of the time we are too tired, too busy, too focussed on other stuff, too sedentary or too tempted - and that's before we've factored in the habit of mindless eating or levels of addiction. When we do things that continually fly in the face of something we believe we want... it's often referred to as "unconscious behaviour". Sometimes it's unconscious because even though we know we're doing it, we simply can't seem to stop ourselves. The short term desire exerts too great a pull - like an undertow we can't control. Other times the "unconscious" part is all of the who where when of the above that we haven't taken on board, let alone reckoned on its combined effect.

To be honest, I don't have an issue with a few pounds here and there. It's chickenfeed, though keeping a few pounds in check does keep your eye on the ball as well as providing a safety net, some window for movement. But when it's the beginning of a slippery slope that can end up putting life and health out of balance and no longer feeling in charge of ourselves, then it's worth a look.

This is about getting Back in Charge as well as Balancing the Scales.

Let's zoom in, take a closer look, and begin to get sorted!!

It ain't just the food!!
A Look at Social & Emotional Eating Behaviours

Anyone familiar with fighting the flab will have tried and tested a myriad of diets over the years, but seeing's most of us aren't daft as well as overweight... how come we fall down the same hole... again, and again? Clearly, *what* we are eating – *is* fundamental, but why and when is often overlooked yet belongs just as firmly in the weight loss / weight holding - at the right end of the scales - equation. Establishing then how and why we repeat the same old eating behaviours is the one thing which will throw light on the most effective way of dealing with it. In many ways it's no different to budgeting with money: we'll spot the big layouts, like holidays, prioritize the essentials – i.e. rent, mortgage etc, come what may, yet somehow give short shrift to off the cuff treats... and yet it adds up.

We eat primarily to function physically - to maintain body temperature and keep active and survive. But we also eat to provide meaning and structure to our lives 365 days a year, to pass time, commemorate, celebrate, share with others, or because of life / work / family circumstances: long hours, too tired, too hungry, too late... and that's before we've even taken on board the almost unconscious eating that can take place when we're upset, stressed, bored, whatever... and not even actually hungry. And overeating as a reaction to negative emotion or prolonged fatigue can make it incredibly difficult to maintain resolve or dietary moderation. Add self recrimination to the pile and reaching out for more edible or liquid comfort becomes a firmly entrenched cycle, a way of muddling through which then hardens into habit - and bad habits really are the barnacles on the bottom of the boat. My job is to help you spot them, weed them out and replace them with good ones.

At its most over-simplistic, there's situational overeating and there's emotional overeating, but if you drew a line with one at each end, most of us would be somewhere along that line and less commonly at one extreme or the other.

What's common to many overeaters though is that point when our hardly noticeable slip slide up the scales seems to accelerate, all of an apparent sudden, into the fat equivalent of negative compound interest (aka escalating credit card!) – that veering out of control, more than the sum of the parts weight gain.

Two of the things I hear most frequently when people have been trying to lose weight, carry on losing weight past the inevitable plateau, or more poignantly put it all back on again is that they are "so good all day until they get home," and that they do know what to do, if only they could "stick to it."

Obviously there are many variations but our capacity for sabotaging our best efforts almost within hours or days, continually undermining whatever we were so sure we could do, is rather like having a car with unreliable brakes: very dodgy, very upsetting, very unsafe, and weight and physical health aside, not feeling that we can rely on ourselves, losing our sense of personal accountability, slowly but surely corrodes our self esteem.

Being in charge of our decision making and actions, at least more often than not, is essential to our wellbeing. Losing that control becomes a kind of bottom line deal breaker. And then to crown it we get fat. So what could possibly be so hard? How come we can keep to our word perfectly well in other areas of our lives, but fall so short with modifying our eating behaviour?

So recognizing what's going on, yer eating behaviour mojo, is really pivotal to the plot!! While it may seem to demand more time than you're willing to give, if weight related issues are taking up a whole lot of your mental and emotional space anyway, it's a worthy investment!! Rather like learning something new, it initially takes the focus but eventually becomes second nature…

A word to the wise:
Throughout everything, all of your efforts, the one thing you have to really make sure of is that whatever diet or revised eating plan you choose, it **has to work for you,** enough, over time. It absolutely **has to be sustainable.** The use of the word "diet" nowadays generally implies a reduction of our intake from the moderate to the dramatic. It is simply a

more extreme version of "sensible eating" to get to us to the same place faster. We do it instead of the sensible eating, because we believe the reward of quicker weight loss has half a hope of overriding our waning willpower, or whatever else gets in the way. And this **can** work well. But whatever we do **has to** be followed with something which is **different** to what we did before, otherwise, no surprise here, we get back what we had before. Establishing a regime to follow on from whatever diet we have followed, puts into place a "way of being" which guides and contains you, while allowing for life and enjoyment to exist within it!! Moreover, it rests more workably between the extremes of over dieting or overeating. In other words it is sustainable over time, for the most part.

Dieting as a bridge toward a new regime
= successful weight holding.

I labour the point because it is so absolutely fundamental, but I will provide you with ways to put this in place in the Tricks of the Trade chapter later on.

Leaping past the wisdom of conventional dieting and sufficient activity however, I will help you unpick exactly what is going on before any dieting even begins. None of this is rocket science but if it were simply a matter of eating "sensibly" we'd have done it. The thing we are dealing with here over and above calorie intake and nutritional education is a combination of **lifestyle situations** and circumstance over which you may or may not have control; the need for **emotional or physical comfort**, which is anything derived from eating in reaction to an emotion, to eating because we are overtired or hormonal or whatever; the effect of **thought and beliefs** on our actions and its influence on how we see things, and the **power of habit** in binding the whole lot together and keeping us well and truly stuck.

This Gang of Four are a powerful set of bedfellows. And assuming willpower alone hasn't worked for you else you wouldn't be here, we're going to get to know how and where and when they appear on your personal map. This will become your **Eating Behaviour Blueprint.** As I reiterate throughout, in any other aspect of your lives, particularly if it related to your children, or your work, you wouldn't keep barking up the same tree if it proved fruitless. You'd check what was going on and shift your strategy. That's what we'll be doing here.

Out of the Out of Awareness... box... and...
... getting to know your Eating Behaviour Blueprint.

The main aim in this book is to make plain the obvious and discover the not so obvious: to name areas you may be familiar with but hadn't factored in or reckoned on sufficiently. On the basis that whatever you've been doing hasn't been working well enough, or is floundering too much of the time, we'll be going back through these areas for an in depth look to see what could have been missed. Checking what it is that for you, comprises "overeating" and seeing where and how and when all of this could be happening. What are the trigger areas, or circumstances, both predictable and unpredictable, that can lead astray and pile on the pounds. What are the underlying emotions, and how your physical wellbeing comes into the equation. Assuming you are motivated and ready, which we'll also be looking at, recognition is crucial.

The second main step is to take a look at the nature of habit, and where it gets a hold.

Most of us when we diet, are trying to undo eating habits by virtue of calorie reduction or changing what we eat, changing what we do as a norm, whilst leaving in place... the habits that keep these in place!! And since a well grounded habit lives, as it is designed, largely out of awareness, in our unconscious, like an automatic pilot operating behind the scenes, the first step here is to at least become aware of what is going on and when. If you believe you are already aware, then it might be about turning up the volume. It is almost impossible to change something, or to make that change last, (i.e. holding the weight once you get there) if we don't know what the odds are, or what's lying in wait to sabotage our best attempts!! Often it's the battle in our heads that puts the cat amongst the pigeons, the negative assumptions or variations on "I've blown it" or "It's not fair" that mark the slippery slope downhill. Other times it's the circumstances of our lives that leave us little time or space to think, let alone to plan for our wellbeing. But most times it's a mix of both to some degree or other. So we'll be fine tooth combing areas of your lives and the things you do, the places you go and the people who share your environment. This will form the basis of your personal map: the blueprint that is unique to you. In this respect, as in any forensic quest, the details specific to you and you alone are paramount. Generalities tell us how we are all similar, and all of us have extra weight due to too much taken in or too little burnt off or the wrong kind of foods. The map you'll be putting together will be your personal blueprint; the DNA of your *own* relationship with food. Not someone else's. This alone will help you through.

Finally, in as practical and common sense a way as possible, looking at how the habits can be undone, or overridden. Starting always with the easiest and working up from there. On the basis that the most challenging points will more likely be a work in progress for the duration, we'll leave those till last! Sometimes that's to do with where you are in your life right now: a working mum may have her work cut out with long hours and a lot of demand on her personal time whereas a mum at home may have too much time near the kitchen. A person living alone could have too much time to do what they please, and eat what they please - and that's before taking on board the whole spectrum of emotional factors.

The entire book may not be a wand, but it can have a magical effect on your understanding, your perspective, and hence your ability to make change, and moreover, change that lasts. As in maintaining a healthier weight and out of the eternal yo-yoing change. It will highlight a lot of what you know already, and bring into awareness a lot of stuff you'd either forgotten or hadn't thought of , which added into the equation, adds that last piece to the jigsaw. The jigsaw is the full picture, rather than a part picture, of what is really going on. Having the full picture means you are better informed to make better choices, and put insight into action. Action that lasts.

* * *

Looking at ourselves through history, it can't help but be mused that the human spirit seems to excel in times of adversity and lack, but that we ain't so hot at managing ongoing excess.

Testimony to this are the myriad of religious teachings which cautioned against the paths of temptation, and the number of highly evolved Masters themselves who struggled to rise above it. We forget that *real* freedom is not simply being allowed to "taste the forbidden", but to be able to stop, or moderate, when we choose. Being able to act on this choice – is what actually sets us free.

Mastery over desire, be it love of food, drink, cigarettes, drugs, shopping, gambling, love, sex, money, power... is common to us all in some form, but is also something we usually only bother with once the cost of our enjoyment or whatever we get out of it... runs out of control, and is costing us, emotionally or financially or physically or spiritually... far, far more than any benefit provided at the outset, but somehow cannot now be stopped. The negative impact is now offsetting any pleasure by a distance, but we are stuck, and the tail is definitely wagging the dog.

* * *

On the upside... is the relative expertise and wealth of dietary and nutritional knowledge many of you will have accumulated from all the years of trying!

It means you're getting started on terrain you already know and much as it might feel like starting all over, you never, ever go back to square one. It's *not* a revolving door but rather a grandly spiralling staircase, which means that every now and then you are at a similar position to where you first began, but higher up, and with a much better perspective. Please hold to that thought as well, when you feel like you're getting nowhere...

So, on this basis:

Some of you will be supremely skilled at Weight *Gain...* with some excelling more than others.

Many of you will be exceptionally skilled at Weight *Loss* even if it's for short bursts of time.

What we all want is to become highly skilled at Weight *Holding*, at the right end of the scales.

To do this we need *all* of the jigsaw pieces, not just the one about "Diets".

The complete jigsaw is your entire personal map of all your lifestyle and circumstantial and emotional eating behaviours combined. It also comes with the hidden bits, called "Habit", which will need your perseverance and curiosity ideally to keep going till you get it. It's like operating behind the scenes, with a blindfold, but it's a crucial part of the overall game plan.

Getting slim and staying slim and staying healthy and all it means to each of you is not merely a process of getting light. It can be a process of absolute enlighten*ment*!

So HOW COME WE OVEREAT?
A brief overview of the big picture:

Over and above keeping us warm and providing energy, eating adds structure to our day and socially, it adds meaning to our lives. It provides a framework within which we work and play and sleep.

I refer to this as the social spectrum - but it's the sum total of our lifestyles with its situations and events and schedules. In its own right it is already challenging enough to manage the many options for eating more than we need but at least it is visible.

Conversely, emotional eating can be a trickier customer. Less easy to pin down and far more resistant to the kind of willpower we use in other areas, we may or may not be conscious of just how much we do this, but most of us do it to some extent.

Essentially then, there's social overeating, which is heavily **time** and **event** related, and there's emotional overeating, bearing in mind that this is anything we eat when not actually hungry and which is surplus to physical requirement. Of course they don't operate alone, and one almost invariably affects the other, but if you drew a line with one at each end, most of us would be somewhere along that line and less commonly at one extreme or the other.

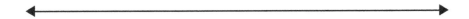

Social   *Emotional*

Obvious as it may be, the idea in separating them out is so that we can more easily recognise how things start and what lies beneath our overeating. When we can actually see what is going on we are far more likely to make better choices in how we manage things: recognition is absolutely the first step and by doing this you are already making a difference, you are already doing something. As I reiterate throughout, if it were that simple, we'd have done it. We'd be masters of moderation and there'd be no obesity crisis.

Even if the overload of calories is initially driven by that hamster wheel of lifestyle plus work, the sum total of too much to do in too little time, the picking at bits or going for the most easily available fast food reaction is still a hard nut to break and if your "habit" wasn't emotionally driven to begin with, frustration and upset or disappointment often make it so by the end.

Many people do however describe themselves as emotional eaters and notice reaching for food as a reaction to stress, yet may still not appreciate just how strong a hold this has until they try to moderate their eating, or until they try to maintain the weight loss they've achieved. The fact that 90% of people who lose weight regain it within 6 to 12 months is testimony to this. While habit can be blamed, there is a world of difference between a repeated reflex action - like reaching for a light switch in its old place after moving house - and trying to stop something which has emotional tenterhooks more deeply embedded in your unconscious. Speaking from personal experience it's rather like giving up cigarettes: long after the nicotine has left your body and years after the reflex of hand to mouth for a puff has subsided, you can still have that vestige of longing at moments of intense stress. No such longing however, remains for the light switch!

It is precisely that longing which drives the repeated action. The nature of the compulsion and what sets it off is key, it is your way through. Even if your eating is less apparently emotional and more about succumbing over and again to temptation, see how you feel when you attempt to cut out the extras. If you are 85% or more in charge of yourself in this respect, you are unlikely to have purchased this book. So it's worth looking back at your success rate in managing your eating as an indication of where you are on the "Habit" scale. Rather like doing yearly accounts, this is about taking stock so that you get an increasingly clear idea of the full picture. It is no different to budgeting.

Again, a line used to denote a continuum can be useful to pinpoint where you might be on a spectrum from low level habit, to high level habit. Low level habit indicating a greater success rate in curbing habitual eating behaviours leading to weight gain, and high level habit being the exact opposite.

Low level habit   *High level habit*

Finally, the bit that was too long to fit in the title of the book but is an essential piece of the jigsaw – is **PHYSICALLY driven overeating**. I will cover this later, but in nutshell form it is this:

If you are tired an awful lot of the time, whether that is due to ill health, pain, or more commonly not sleeping well enough or long enough, the first thing that tends to diminish is your focus and resolve. Apart from glucose levels dropping and a greater susceptibility to sugars and processed carbs, that one factor alone can increase emotional volatility on some level or other and the likelihood of treat or comfort eating. I mention this because the incidence of people being tired beyond belief yet wondering why on earth they cannot curb a simple overeating habit which is piling on the pounds, is incredibly high. And of course tiredness can both arise from, and impact, socially or emotionally driven eating behaviours. It's negatively self reinforcing:

| **Social / Situational Lifestyle** | **Physically driven overeating e.g. tiredness / pain etc** | **Emotional overeating** |

Time & event related

Ultimately, assuming you have been trying over and again to manage your eating yet somehow default at the first sight or smell of temptation, then there is a **gap between what you planned to do and what you ended up doing.** Or put differently, a gap between the original intention and the eventual behaviour, and you are filling that gap with food or drink. Whether the difference between what you planned and what you actually did is due to too much temptation, too little sleep, too little head space, emotional issues, or a fab combo of any or all of those, this is what we need to explore. Understanding and becoming aware of what is going on in that gap is your key to more successfully managing eating patterns and behaviours. It allows us to nourish and "feed" ourselves in a way which better serves the purpose. The more you are able to do this, the less urgent the compulsion to eat or drink. Sometimes it's a matter of just slightly reducing the tipping point. There's always a tipping point.

Intention   **Behaviour**
What you planned to do   **What you ended up doing"**

MINDING THE GAP!

8 am   **7 pm**
Begin diet today   **"I'll start tomorrow"**

Remember, however much you know this, and you do, the bit we have yet to know better and get a hold of is the part of us come tea time or whenever, that still decides to do something entirely different yet repeatedly regrets it the following morning! What we need to understand better are the tripwires which catch us out between what we mean to do, at the one end, and what we end up doing, at the other.

Some of where we need to look springs from old behaviours, entrenched habits, ways of thinking and how we see things, and other times it's food and temptation itself. I refer to this as Tracing the Roots and Trigger Tracking.

Put the lot together and it's a minefield of tripwires. The detective work is tracking those tripwires, throwing light on them, and creating strategies to cope.

Tracking the tripwires: team mates of the Gang of Four

Although I cover the contents of the next couple of pages in far greater depth throughout the book, I want to at least sew the ideas prior to the issue of whether you actually need to lose weight, whether you are ready, and so on. Hopefully this not so subtle weaving in and out will filter through and properly hit the spot by the time I ask you to start collecting evidence. (Yes, you'll be collecting evidence!)

- Temptation. It tastes so good. We can resist anything but temptation.

- Emotional compensation. Food comforts, it rewards, it treats, etc etc.

- Physical and hormonal. Difficult to hold resolve when tired... etc.

- Habit. Do the same thing enough times, and you do it... just because...

- Lifestyle. Too little time or too much time, too much structure, too little structure, doing what you love, or stuck in what you don't, it all adds up...

- Ineffective goal setting and prioritizing. Not recognizing what stops us.

- Perspective and negative thinking. It's not what you see but how you see it. Letting negative self talk undo a mountain of great work. Head in the sand denial and variations of "I've blown it".

Recognition is the key.

What gets in the way? Glitches in the M.O...

If you think about it, the capacity for millions of us, en masse, to fall off a diet and then put weight back on again is actually quite a phenomenon. It would be funny, if it weren't so massively frustrating and such a head banging waste of time. In most areas we are more than capable of setting an intention and holding to it, and if it doesn't come to pass – we've usually had a choice in the matter or at least we have a sense of why.

Somehow, in the area of eating behaviours, the gap between what we mean to do and what we end up doing has quite a wide divide. The statement of the obvious is that although we think we know what we want, some other part of us at varying points down the line and with varying frequency... is wanting something different. It's our failure to take this on board and surprise at the inevitable outcome which is perhaps more intriguing.

Because of this extraordinary phenomenon, this expertise in falling down the same hole, again and again, specifically, I'm going to briefly unpick the process of wanting something and what might be in the way of getting it and holding on to it. While you're reading this, maybe keep in mind your dieting history and see if it makes more sense.

1 – Needing to prioritize elsewhere: life etc... gets in the way...

There's a lot of things we all want which don't necessarily end up happening, even when we want them badly: lack of opportunity, circumstance i.e. time money etc, and other more important things which demand our attention. No mystery there. Sometimes it's genuine, sometimes it's procrastination, as below, but other times we may not take on board just how much we are stuck on the hamster wheel of "stuff" which has no place overriding our core needs. Often this goes hand in hand with putting ourselves last, (Mums!) and needing to recognise that our emotional and physical wellbeing actually has an impact on those around us.

2 – Procrastination

Can be similar to the above… but to clarify…

Most of us have stuff we really, really want to do because it brings us something meaningful, but somehow in the day to dayness of things always gets put off till tomorrow, which of course never comes. There are varying reasons for putting things off, which may include:

a) Not believing them to have the same importance as something more immediately essential.

b) Believing we don't have the time. This may or may not be actually true, over time, and may be either realised consciously, or buried somewhere out of view, hence unconscious. Life, stuff, general debris and other habits get in the way. You feel you "ought" to fit it in but don't, or believe you can't.

c) Fearing we won't get it right and will fail anyway, so (distorted thinking here) why start at all.

3 – Not enough fuel for lift off and lasting the course…

Other times the level of wanting something passes or doesn't hold sufficient interest in the first place, both to propel us into action and to sustain that action over time.

Other than circumstance and just drifting (into careers, relationships, lifestyles…) it's generally passion or urgency that makes us take one direction or another which I refer to as *honeymoon* or *emergency motivation.* Whether it's a sudden decision or something you've been considering a while, there's going to be a tipping point, a level of sufficiency as it were, in terms of the energy needed for the desire to take shape and get lift off. I call this energy your motivating "fuel". Otherwise it's just a whim.

4 – Getting and Goal Setting…

Again, no real mystery, when something becomes extremely important to us, we create the conditions for it to take place. Often this is incredibly automatic and there's just a natural prioritising toward a particular end.

We consciously look at anything which could get in the way and factor it in. Even when we have more than one pressingly important goal, we're either able to accommodate that, or one has to take precedence over another. So what goes awry...?

5 – Conflicting goals and unconscious prioritizing.....

This in effect is when we are at odds with ourselves, but it is not always obvious that what we want is conflicting with something else. It's happening almost behind the scenes, in our blind spot. Other times it is obvious but we don't know what to do about it. Trying for example to moderate what you eat with a permanently full house and a full time job and you are the main cook... has your work cut out from the start. It's challenging enough with full awareness not to let our focus slip elsewhere, but when we don't take all the factors on board it's a virtual non starter... It is exactly because this is so par for the course, because we are all constantly juggling so many different aspects of our lives, that we need to appreciate the combined impact of social and emotional issues: these are what make it grist for the mill and which I go into in depth later on.

6 – Levels of Motivation: lack of recognition and insight...

Possibly one of the biggest pitfalls other than underestimating the power of habit is the failure to differentiate between levels of motivation. We tend to assume that the motivation which accompanies a wake up call of some kind with its rocket launching impetus, will somehow continue. Surely if we want something enough, which is a fair enough assumption given how much effort we've put in to achieving our goals, and the hard time we give ourselves when we continually fall off the wagon...surely our resolve would match our desire. You'd think... But what needs factoring in is the intensity of our early need which is what I call *emergency motivation,* and *motivation over time.* They characterize the difference between losing weight, and holding weight, and will usually need a *different approach.*

6b ... followed by need for humour and self compassion...

We tend to make two errors of judgement: the first is in not realising that it's perfectly natural and in the order of things for the intensity of the initial motivation to wane. The second is to berate ourselves for lack of willpower which far from inspiring a move for the better tends to deplete what remaining reserves we have. And for anyone who eats to console, guess what happens? Yep, we eat something to make ourselves feel better for failing in our quest not to eat whatever we eat in the way we do. A beautiful kind of mini insanity, a mental disorder for the normally sane. This however is where it is seriously important to have a sense of humour. Funny it may not be, in essence, but there is something kinda crazy about how we operate, and seeing as another dose of shame will most likely incur another dose of compensatory snacking, the humour – otherwise known in this case as self compassion, seems the better option... surely?

7 – Different types of "wanting": genuine desire v impulse and habit! "I can resist anything but temptation"...

Ok this is the biggie: other than the stuff of circumstance and all of the above, the main "conflicting goal" when it comes to food, which unlike cigarettes or alcohol, we need to stay alive so cannot avoid, is dieting itself. Assuming you haven't gained weight because you are immobilised or medicated, the task most of us have is to get a grip on what is generically, reactive eating. The problem is that a lot of the time, whether it's emotional or circumstantial, "impulse based wanting" has its own rocket fuel. Depending on how and why and what it stems from will dictate its level of demand, but it has a nasty little grip and what comes to mind is the rapidly growing cactus in "The Little Shop of Horrors" musical, whose incessant cry of "Feed me Rocky, feed me!!" became as creepy as it was funny.

Dieting is *in itself a conflicting goal!* So this is getting to be like one of those board games which looks easy to start but in fact, the more you wade in, the more there are complications! Staving off all the wonderfully rewarding or delaying or anaesthetizing effects of impulse eating on a daily basis in order to achieve an end which is way in the distance, has to be the ultimate challenge in delaying gratification. And a lot of the problem is needing to stay fully alert to those impulses, 18/7 if not 24/7. (By the way this is why the Alternate Day diet[1], or variations of, can work such a treat, as at least you're not gagging at the bit for months and can see an end in sight on a 24 to 48 hour basis in terms of temporary relief, whilst still being on track.....)

People invariably ask what they can do to counteract the lasso pull of the unexpected impulse. Becoming increasingly familiar with where and when they occur, which we'll be going through in the next few chapters, is already a first step. When we observe something it means it's no longer hidden out of awareness and so takes away some of its power. The other step is being crystal clear about what it is you're going for and knowing you want it 100 per cent. That 100 per cent will provide the willingness to look out for your areas of least resistance (impulses) and either sidestep them or factor them in, in a way which keeps them at bay. (See "Lighting your Fire and other distractions" later on.)

8 – Not really knowing what you want and what it will do for you...

You can see how, in order to withstand the massive pull of temptation and being sidetracked on a daily basis, you have to be even more tempted by the end product and what that holds for you. You have to be sure enough of what you want and willing enough to give it the attention it needs. Again it isn't right or wrong or good or bad. It's basic law of energy except in this case the energy is your motivation fuel. It's either there or it isn't.

---

[1] The Alternate Day Diet: James B Johnson MD & Donald R Laub Sr MD

Collecting the Evidence: Your Detective In Action
(and keeping a policeman's notebook....!)

It will have become clear from page one that Overeating Unplugged is not about food, bar a short episode on food wisdom... but about eating behaviours, and what keeps them in place, or enables change...

It's main purpose however is to enable each of you to become your own best private investigator, so the trail of crumbs you'll be following, the case you'll be on, is your own. Which means, as I mentioned earlier, you'll be collecting evidence!

Because I have noticed over the years that where there is temptation there is also a very selective memory, I have found it useful to suggest a portable, pocket sized, memory aid. It doesn't matter too much whether it's your phone or a notebook, but it does work better if it is permanently on your person!

If the notebook isn't on you it is highly likely you won't get around to recording the thought, or the event, and whilst it isn't hard to remember something on the same day, it's a different matter as things pile up over the weeks, to record them with any accuracy.

What's it *for* then?....

Its purpose is very specific, very short and very simple: any particular emotions, feelings, that come up, especially the type that suddenly have you chomping at the bit as you pass Costa's, MacDonald's, your local bakery or the food cupboard... write in the date, time of day, climate, place, followed by the feeling, i.e. happy/sad/angry/upset etc etc, and what preceded it or what is coming up. No more, no less. Should you choose to write reams and find the hours have whiled away, that's fine, but the risk is that by day three you might feel you've got better things to do with your time and then not do it at all. By keeping it short it takes a matter of seconds and you're less likely to begrudge the effort. Further, it's going to be a lot easier at a later stage to cast an eye over the material to scan for any patterns. That's why I call it a policeman's notebook – precise, to the point, and easy to refer back to.

The beauty, if I may refer to it as such, of this exercise is twofold: firstly, any patterns which we may not have noticed or thought of before in our eating habits, will suddenly jump up from the page. You might have a feeling that you always get major munchies at a time in the month or when your mother has made yet another timely comment about some aspect of your life... but there's little as convincing as seeing it in black and white. Hard evidence is indisputable, and to the extent that you may have been kidding yourself about elements of your relationship with food, or in denial, seeing it written in front of you has a somewhat sobering effect. Moreover it consolidates the links between lifestyle, emotions and eating behaviours that this book works with throughout.

Should you fill a note book, date it, and keep it somewhere safe: it's your eating behaviour **blueprint!** Above all though, be curious, and have fun!

... if you have time to eat it, you have time to write it...!!

Smoking Yo-yo dieters!! Alert!!
Although this is all about our eating habits, it can be used equally for anything we do to excess and which is having an adverse effect.

As many may have experienced, smoking is often not only an appetite suppressant, (until it isn't..!) but more pertinently fills the same gaps as emotional eating. Use of cigarettes to fill an emotional gap or as a social habit is no different to use of food in that way.

Because of both the return of a good appetite as **much** as the space left from stopping, there is an overwhelming link between giving up smoking and weight gain. Basically it's a swap over. You've simply exchanged one gap filling emotional snug rag for another.

Because of this too, I would encourage anyone who is smoking to notice if the number of cigarettes a day increases when you are trying to eat less and lose weight. Notice and *make note of* the time and the place and with whom. Exactly the same as with overuse of food and drink.

Otherwise the smoking just gets replaced by more food again when you stop your diet and the weight gain seesaw will just keep tipping from one side to the other.

YOUR BEST WEIGHT...
and
DO YOU NEED TO LOSE WEIGHT?

What IS your Best Weight and do you NEED to Lose Weight?

Clients often ask what is the right weight for them and how much they need to lose. Ideal measurements apart, it's worth bearing in mind that *feeling* overweight may not be the same as being overweight, and that if you do have a lot to lose, just starting is the way to go. Telling someone in the morbid obese range that they have to lose 10 stone plus, however obvious, can be paralyzing and waylay the best of intentions. Besides which, if someone has been very obese for a long time they may have little to no reference for gauging where to aim for. By contrast if you've put on a stone or two over many years and are harking back to your more youthful weight, this might be wholly unrealistic by the time you've reached middle age.

Varying factors will influence our concept of "the perfect weight" including our cultural and generational backgrounds and so it is important to separate our notion of attractive, which is highly subjective and very personal, from optimal health.

The facts:
The main guidelines are body mass index (BMI), more currently the waist to hip ratio (WHR) and body fat percentage.

BMI has until recently been used to determine a healthy weight range, with the outer limits being underweight below 18.5 to overweight from 25 upward, and obesity being defined at 30 plus. Calculated by dividing your current weight in kilos, by your height in metres squared, it is still good as a tool for rough screening but what it doesn't take into account is a person's body fat content: this is now seen as a more accurate indicator of future health risks. Added to this are significantly higher levels of glucose and cholesterol in certain ethnicities including those of Chinese and South Asian origin, who should not take a low BMI as an indicator of their health[2].

---

[2] The Heart.org 27/01/2013 and The American Heart Association 22/01/2013 both show "overweight" related symptoms at BMI 21 for the Chinese and 23 for

Central obesity – sometimes called the apple shape - is when you are carrying too much fat around your middle and it is this measurement which is most greatly associated with high cholesterol levels, diabetes type 2, cardiovascular disease, strokes, cancer and even dementia. This is calculated by dividing your waist measurement by your hip measurement and should ideally be no greater than 0.85 for women and 1.0 for men. A much easier way to work it out and remember though is to keep your waist circumference to less than half your height.

Body fat percentage is similar but is more generalized by taking your age, height and weight, gender and waist measurement into account. For our bodies to function well it is essential that they contain a healthy amount of fat to regulate temperature, to insulate our organs and to store energy. Carrying too little means we deprive our bodies of stored energy and begin to use muscle protein as fuel... carrying too much can increase the health risks already mentioned.

These then are the main measurement tools, but how do we feel about our weight?

Feelings and Self Perception:

As a Londoner with a French mother and more vanity than I care to admit, I just love slim. Ok it's a middle of the road BMI 22 but I love feeling elegant enough to carry off a broad range of clothes, I love feeling fit, and I love how it looks on others. *However,* and it's a big however, it's not up to me to burden those others with my concept of attractiveness. That job is already overly accomplished to a ridiculous degree by the media with which our everyday lives are so mercilessly assaulted. So the only real reference with regard to a person's best weight will always be their state of health. Good health cuts across a plethora of agendas – wherever you come from, it's being well and feeling well that counts.

So where do the waters get murky? Self image and how we believe we

---

South Asians. In particular the dramatic rise in type 2 diabetes and early coronary heart disease in South Asians in the Western world, as high as 20% suggest an interaction between genetic disposition and environmental factors.

are seen has a powerful effect on our self esteem. While our uniqueness is highly valued, we are still very tribal in many respects: there is still a level of belonging, of being accepted, that lurks somewhere in the psyche, even if it's well hidden. It's part of our survival make up. And while it's good to shine, standing out from the crowds and being conspicuous for the wrong reasons is not so fun.

Identity with our peers...

Influenced by trends our concept of slim is far more extreme than in say the fifties. Marilyn Monroe and her ilk were often dramatically hourglass but none the less voluptuous. Fast forward to the sixties and Twiggy and Biba led a generation into the new more androgynous petite. Fast forward further and hollow cheeked emaciation has the look, the almost anorexic requirement for dancers and jockeys having spread through the ranks. Currently a justifiable concern for any parent dieting is the impact on an already impressionable teenager, now affecting children as young as five[3]. In fact the curiously skewed effects of eating behaviours resulting in opposing ends of the weight spectrum must surely raise questions even if no conclusions can be drawn: preoccupation with weight and appearance manifesting in ever younger pre pubescent children at the one end, while our susceptibility to excess clearly visible with rising obesity statistics at the other. What this means is that often a person's *idea* of what they would like is at odds with what is both achievable and sustainable for them: this works against us when our sense of failure at not having achieved a particular weight, even just pounds off the mark, starts to affect our eating behaviours: "I've blown it" – surely the most fattening thought process around - seems far more frequently to elicit a kind of "oh well, now I've started..." or "in for a penny, in for a pound" eating reaction than any hoped for moderation. Since this usually occurs at quite an

---

[3] The Guardian 01/08/2011 Susan Greenwood, chief exec of the eating disorders charity B-eat, told the Sunday Telegraph that the figures reflected "alarming" trends in society, with young children "internalising" messages from celebrity magazines, which idealised the thinnest figures.

unconscious, automatic level, it's a great example of where thoughts and feelings affect the very behaviour we're trying to control. It's also then a pointer at what needs addressing before we even think of doing a diet.

Identity and family tradition...
A contrasting example of "out of awareness" thought and eating behaviour reactions can be when a person's idea of the weight they want is at odds with where they come *from*. Second generation ethnicity in particular can elicit an almost extraordinary conflict between ideology and behaviour – where for instance the aspired weight of a woman in a modern, professional, western environment is in conflict with a community which sees weight as a mark of wellness and affluence. To anyone unaffected by this, it might seem an obvious case of making a choice based on preference. Yet the majority of us grossly underestimate the phenomenal effect of background and belief, thought and feelings, on behaviour: one of my clients, an East Caribbean lady in her thirties, could not understand why all her best efforts to obtain a slimness in line with the other women in the city based PR company where she worked, were so thwarted. But returning to her first generation mum and gran and aunts each weekend was having a powerfully negating effect. It wasn't just a case of anything they were saying, far more a question of identity. "This is where I belong. This is how my clan look. This is our tradition." A kind of good to have weight versus be slim to be cool war, raging around her unconscious and playing havoc with her eating plans.

Even minus the ethnic variation, if your family or your peers are mostly overweight due to eating patterns and drinking behaviours, doing something different can be challenging. Though much more in evidence with teenagers, every community has its "norms", and when we veer away from that norm, through what we do or how we appear, that old survival need to fit in with the crowd (adaptation and assimilation) kicks in again: even if our attempt to be healthy isn't taken as a rejection of that crowd, (though surprising how often it is...) the point is it can *feel* that way and act itself out without our understanding why.

What starts to become clear is that before we go anywhere, recognising what lies behind how we'd like to look, whether there are conflicting values or whether all is in harmony, will make a difference in controlling the behaviour we're already working hard to moderate!

Coming full circle, whatever those around you might say, however much they might be put out by a revised eating and drinking plan that's more restrictive, or however awkward you might feel even if they say little, it's a lot easier if you take your health as the yardstick. In the South Asian community for example, there has been such a significant increase in diabetes and heart problems that an unfortunate combination of Western diet together with a genetic disposition for high cholesterol, has to be the main culprit – no doubt McDo' and pizzas and chapattis and rice finally hitting the overload button...[4]

So whether your family and circle of friends and workmates have a culture of over drinking or over eating or simply a preponderance for fat saturated take aways, canapé snacking and fast high heat barbecues – it might seem boring to hold back but not if your health is at stake. What weight is *best* for you and whether you *need* to lose weight should be dictated first and foremost by the health risks posed by a combination of your BMI, your body fat percentage, and your cholesterol levels along with any other symptoms you might experience.

Of course your desire to look good and get into a particular size jeans or dress may be the strongest motivator, and if it is then that is the ball you should run with. But health is the neutral yardstick across race and class, age and fashion.

---

[4] The Heart.org 27/01/2013 and The American Heart Association 22/01/2013 both show "overweight" related symptoms at BMI 21 for the Chinese and 23 for South Asians. In particular the dramatic rise in type 2 diabetes and early coronary heart disease in South Asians in the Western world, as high as 20% suggest an interaction between genetic disposition and environmental factors.

HOW READY ARE YOU?
Your Eating Behaviour Questionnaire

HOW READY ARE YOU?

Most diets work if you stick to them; it's what you do during and after that counts.

For success and long lasting results, any weight loss eating plan has to have a lifestyle and way of being that supports it. It has to be holistic.

Floundering half way or perpetually yo-yoing back up the scales means something's out of synch. What you eat is an essential part of the picture, but it's not the whole story.

The questions that follow are to help you see the whole picture, get it in perspective, and flag up where change is needed. You might be tempted to simply read through at first but if you feel you have a long held problem with overeating and your weight, I'd really encourage you to give yourself the time to fill it in. Even if you come back to it later!

History...

- Have you dieted before?
- How often?
- From what age?
- What's the most you've lost?
- Over what length of time?
- When was your last diet?
- Did you lose as much as you planned?
- How long did you maintain the weight you achieved?

Awareness and recognition...

- When you have stopped diets, whether or not you reached target, have you tended to go straight back to how you ate before?
- Would you describe both what you eat, as well as how much and how often, as being more than you need so contributing to weight gain?
- Describe your general pattern of weight gain – is it:

31

- Slow, pound by pound but over the months.
- Slow at first, but then increasing to a speedy weight gain at the end.
- Fast from shortly after you stopped your dieting.

- Were you aware of the weight going on?
- Do you know why it went on?
- Have you put weight on after giving up smoking?
- Have you used smoking in the past to suppress overeating?
- Do you tend to take action with regard to weight gain:
  - after 7 to 10lbs approx
  - after 10 – 14lbs approx
  - after 1 – 28lbs approx
  - after 28 – 42lbs approx or more
- Do you fool yourself or go into denial about your eating and weight gain?
- Have your eating habits been easy or hard to change? Give a number with 1 being Easy and 10 being very difficult?
- Would someone you value say the same, or otherwise?

Reasons beneath...
- Are you aware of the eating or drinking habits that caused this?
- Does your overeating or drinking tend to be due to:
  - Social / work / family / cultural expectation
  - Living conditions / environment / where you live
  - Lifestyle
  - Emotional
  - Stress from health, illness, money, relationships, work etc.

- Is there a work based or family based or socially based culture of overeating or over drinking that makes moderation very difficult? Is this on a daily basis, or once or twice a week?

- If your work environment is open plan, is food brought in and offered round / left in sight on desks etc?

- What are the main emotions that trigger your overeating?

  -

  -

  -

- What are the main situations that trigger your overeating?

  -

  -

  -

- Does your overeating get triggered with certain people?

- Do you know why?

- Do you overeat when you are stressed?

- Is your stress more work related or personal?

- Do you overeat when you are bored, or to fill or pass the time?

- For you is boredom:

  - Too much time?

  - Nothing to do?

  - Stuck doing things you don't enjoy?

  - Anything else?

- Do you overeat or drink to put off things you dread doing?

- Do you eat or drink as a reaction to situations or emotions?

  - Some of the time?

  - A lot of the time?

  - Most of the time?

- Do you overeat simply out of habit, when you are not even hungry?
- From 1 to 10, how willing are you to make changes?
- From 1 to 10, how *able* are you to make changes?

When and where...

- Does your overeating entail:
    - Picking in between meals, grazing through the day?
    - "Camel" mindset, i.e. eating for the long haul, worrying you may not get anything later so overfilling in the meantime?
    - Lack of portion control and several helpings?
    - Eating on the run?
    - Eating alone or secret eating?
    - Eating in the car?
    - Going without food for too long then overeating once you do eat?
    - Eating heavily within three hours of going to bed?

Food wisdom...

- Is your eating over high in (the wrong) fats, sugars, processed carbohydrates or starch?
- Do you fry a lot?
- Do you eat take aways:
    - Once a week?
    - Twice?
    - How many times if more?
- Is your main weight gain more through food or drink?
- How many fizzy drinks do you have a day, or a week?
- How much alcohol do you drink a day, or a week?
- Do you notice yourself picking or overeating more after alcohol?

- Would you describe what you eat as:
  - Healthy;
  - Quite healthy;
  - Not at all healthy;
- Irrespective of what you actually do end up eating, would you say your **understanding** of how to eat well, of what makes a healthy, balanced eating plan is:
  - Very good;
  - Quite good;
  - Not good at all.

Structure and timing...

- Do you find you eat or drink more:
  - Some days
  - Week days
  - Weekends
  - Everyday
- What time of the day are you most likely to pick or overeat?
- Do you eat or drink more when you have too much time? I.e. when your time is less structured?
- Do you eat or drink more when you have too little time?
- Do you eat or drink more when your days are too long?
- Do you eat or drink more when you are out of the usual routine?
- Do you eat or drink more when you travel / stay away from home?

Wellbeing...

- Do you eat or drink more when you are tired?
- Do you get enough sleep?

- Do you often feel tired, or under par?
- Is this something you can change? Can you get to bed earlier?
- Does lack of enough activity make it difficult to maintain a healthy weight?
- Is your job mainly sedentary?
- Is your physical mobility restricted for any reason?
- Would you be willing or able to increase your activity in any way: (This can be *any* kind of movement)?
  - By 5 minutes a day?
  - By 15 minutes a day?
  - By 30 minutes a day?
  - By 30 minutes two or three times a week?
- What kind of activity could you do that you don't manage now?
- How and when would you fit it into your day?

Support network...

- Do your friends or family have or understand eating behaviour and weight issues?
- Would friends or family support both weight loss and weight maintenance process?
- Would friends or family support the revised eating plans for *maintaining* your weight loss?
- Do you tend to feel supported or isolated in your weight loss and weight maintenance efforts?
- Does it go against the grain with work or family?
- Are you aware that support is important in keeping the weight off long term?

- Do you have anyone who supports you?
  - Family
  - Partner
  - Friends
  - Work colleagues
  - Professional support i.e. group or counsellor

Different from before…?

- Compared to before what would be different this time?
- Is your mindset or attitude different this time?
- Do you feel more motivated than on previous times?
- Are you open to changing your relationship with food, as well as just dieting?
- How much do you now recognize that keeping the weight off needs as much focus as losing the weight in the first place?
- What have you learnt from previous dieting?
- When you go back to less restricted eating, will this be different from your current eating patterns?
- Do you appreciate that normal eating is not the same as what was previously "normal" for you, if you have described your previous intake as surplus to requirement..? (Apologies for statement of the obvious, but this is *the* tripwire of tripwires… so not so obvious after all…)

How Ready are you this time?

- Are your current circumstances, i.e. life, health, work, personal, conducive to making changes in how and when you eat?
- Is there time and mental space for you to focus on these changes?

- Do you believe you will be able to continue in this way once your target weight, clothes size, or health aims are achieved?
- What might stop you or sabotage you?
- How might you stop or sabotage yourself?

Motivation and meaning...

- What's your top reason for wanting to weigh less than you do now?
- What other areas will benefit from your weight loss and how?
- To what extent do you hope or believe it will change your life for the better:
  - A little – up to 15%
  - Quite a bit – up to 25%
  - Considerably – up to 50%
  - Very much – up to 75%
  - Totally - up to 100%

Notice your feelings and reactions as you read and complete the questionnaire. Anyone who habitually overrides their satiety receptors may also be using food to override emotions, so that until the type or amount of food is taken out of the equation, there may not even be an awareness of doing this: it's become so automatic.

Our emotions however, give us information. I will be encouraging you throughout to notice and observe in a practical way, since these are things we can see and touch and know. There is no mystery, it is easy to collect the "evidence" and because of this it is less fearful. This is where Overeating Unplugged will help you become your own best Private Investigator, except the case you are on, is your own!

As you begin to separate reactive eating from conscious, mindful eating, as you become familiar with your energy levels, you will increasingly have an intuitive sense of what is right for you. Paying heed to this will be your surest guide to regaining a better reference point for future weight holding at the right end of the scales.

Ask yourself:

    What do I *want?*

    What am I *willing* to do?

    What am I *able* to do?

    Am I *ready?*

PART 1:
TRACING THE ROOTS 1

What eating MEANS to you.
Your RELATIONSHIP with FOOD.

To get an increased sense of the part food has played in your life, have a look at the list below. These are many of the things people have said "Food Does for Them" over and above our need to have enough energy, maintain body temperature, and basically stay alive.

Remember none of this is bad, or wrong. It's simply an information gathering exercise: as you read through the list, see what hits base. Notice and tick what sounds like you, and add your own. Then give it an "intensity level" out of 10. As your list grows, what will become obvious is just how much we can feel the rug pulled from under our feet when we suddenly reduce calories or take away our comfort fillers, even if the reduction is going from serious *over*eating to normal. For people whose use of food is a pathological reaction to all emotions and situations, pulling away can feel like a real bereavement. It's the equivalent of cold turkey. It also highlights why anyone considering gastric or bariatric surgery needs not only to understand their relationship with food, but to be able to work with it. Insight and recognition are essential first steps, but the ability to put insight into practice is the magic ingredient. For anything. And that can be a work in progress.

- Food tastes fantastic. It makes me feel good.

- Eating helps me get my brain into gear, and then get on with my day.

- Eating breaks up the working or recreational day, makes it more meaningful.

- Food is a great way to share with people. Eating and drinking together bonds.

- Eating can be sacred, like at bar mitzvahs, Diwali, Christmas etc. It accompanies a ritual and brings us together.

- Eating makes everything worthwhile.

- I eat when I can't have love or sex.

- I overeat so that I keep away love, or sex. My weight becomes a barrier.
- Eating fills the time.
- I eat when I am bored.
- Eating gives me a sense of purpose.
- Eating gives me something to look forward to.
- Food makes me feel better.
- Food is like a friend, or a lover. It's there when I need.
- I overeat when I feel lonely.
- I overeat when I feel upset or sad.
- I overeat when I'd rather have love.
- I enjoy eating with a special person, it gives us something to do and share.
- Eating passes the time.
- I overeat when I am angry.
- Food is a comfort.
- Food is my reward for lots of things: If I've worked hard, been good etc.
- Having lots of food around makes me feel safe.
- I overeat sometimes instead of communicating. Like eating my words.
- Overeating eases pain.
- Eating can numb out other stuff I find difficult or emotionally challenging.
- Eating is something I can do here, now, when I can't have or control other things.
- Eating is like how I feel... often out of control.
- I overeat because I feel ashamed.
- I overeat because I feel stuck, or trapped in a situation.

- I overeat because I feel stuck in my life.

- I overeat because it keeps down all the difficult emotions.

- Eating makes me feel less distressed.

- I overeat because I hate myself.

- I overeat when I need something else even if I'm not sure what that something is.

- I overeat when I am studying, or forced to sit down in one place for some reason.

- I overeat when I have to do paperwork, like my tax forms.

- I eat as a reaction to lots of emotions and situations.

- I overeat when I am depressed.

- I overeat but I don't know why. It's a habit I just can't seem to stop.

- I eat to keep myself fat.

- I eat for the starving millions.

- I eat because I hurt.

- I eat to punish myself.

- I eat to try to control my emotions.

Add any of your own that may not be covered here. You might want to include drinking or smoking. It's the same deal!

-

-

-

-

-

-

-

-

Looking through the ones you've ticked or added in, ask yourself "Is this true?" especially if you've given it a high number out of ten.

For example, if you eat "to make yourself feel better", is this *true*? Does it actually make you feel *better* in the long run? Or even half an hour later?

Ask yourself, "Am I usually pleased with my choice two hours later?"

Also, notice the original "pay off" and ask yourself whether the long term consequences are actually outweighing the benefits, especially if the purpose was to quell a feeling. For example if you overeat when you feel hurt or upset, but now your weight is making you feel even more hurt and upset, flagging that up and highlighting that the function behind your overeating isn't serving its purpose, however unconscious, is going to be the first step forward. And should your heart be sinking, remember, this is not about beating yourself up, which serves zilch, but about collecting information, and noticing. That alone *is* a first step, even if you still can't stop whatever you're doing. Hang in there.

From now on too, if you re-iterate any of the negative statements on the list, **use the past tense,** act **as if it were true in the past, but no longer.** For example "I **used** to eat as a reaction to all emotions," or "I **used** to eat to punish myself." Even if it feels ridiculous, (people often start to laugh...) it's sending a message yet again that you are serious about this. The fact you feel ridiculous at all means you are stopping in your tracks and not just acting unconsciously. A lot of the time, recognition is the foot in the door, the first step to detaching a repeated action from its habitual hidey hole! It's saying, hey you! I'm onto you!! It's like the culprit we're really after is that bit of ourselves that hides in our blind spot. And by the way, **humour,** not pain, or shame, is one of the best ways through. It melts resistance far more effectively than any amount of self reproach and remonstrating. And I'm talking about the humour that stems from compassion and caring rather than the type which nervously deflects from a difficult situation.

Finally, especially if you're someone who knows you're going to have to cut down a lot, and for quite a time, remember you are not having to give up on all of it, and it needn't be forever, though ultimately – you may choose to leave out some types of food if you've managed to abstain for a month or more. There's a difference between a food which is a slight trigger to overeat, and one which has the effect of a Class A drug. In a way it's like a co-dependent relationship. You are both separating for a while – but it's not final. Julia Griggs Havey describes this movingly in her book "The Vice Busting Diet" in which she began her massive descent down the scales simply by omitting ice cream, which at the time of writing at least, she had chosen not to reintroduce as a treat. It is really important to remind yourself every inch of the way – **it is *your* choice. The choice is *always yours.***

Ask yourself always:

"Will I be pleased with my choice in two hours time?"

WHAT DO YOU ACTUALLY WANT?

WHAT DO YOU ACTUALLY WANT?

There are at least 365 reasons a year for tempting you off track or not getting started in the first place. Eating and drinking are great pastimes as well as emotional comforters. So being really clear about what you want and whether it matters enough is essential. Because here is the thing:

"Whatever being a healthier weight, or being slimmer will give you – you have to want it *1% more* than the extra food / drink in front of you, enough of the time."

It's like a seesaw with a bucket at each end. In one bucket is everything you're hoping to achieve and hold on to. In the other is the sum total of all the eating distractions taking you in the opposite direction.

Of course this is the case when you begin your diet, but it applies even *more* once you have your weight down. The annual **MoT** for any "foodie", in my book, equals **Motivation over Time**. It's the bit that we forget as we slip back to what *used* to be normal and yo-yo back up again and as statistically this is 90 per cent of us, it is worth watching out for!! Overeating Unplugged is, in essence, all about how to hold your ground in this respect.

So you have to want what you're aiming for *one tiny bit more* than the temptation immediately in front of you, often enough, to keep the see saw going in the right direction. At any given time, your actions will be taking you towards one direction, or the other, however imperceptibly. Whatever sets you off onto the "wrong direction" will either be so deeply embedded into automatic pilot you hardly notice, or have its own alluring benefits package bidding you come hither! By becoming increasingly conscious of where you habitually renege on the direction you most want, you can begin to make a different choice before the pull is out of your control. The tipping point doesn't just happen all of a sudden and it can be balanced back in your favour, at any time.

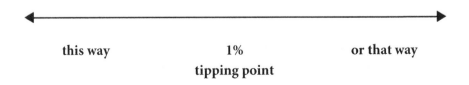

this way	1%	or that way
	tipping point	

Recognising what's important to you will increase your alertness whenever situations threaten to take you off track or impulse strikes, giving you back some choice in the matter. Knowing what you want is what will help you past temptation and override the power of old habits. It's your rocket fuel for lasting success and what you need to get you past first base.

RED ALERT:

Do however reality check and make sure you separate fiction from fact: if what you are hoping for is something you have never experienced, you might want to take a good hard look at whether the possibility holds true.

Believing that "becoming thin" will solve all your life's problems, or bring you happiness or confidence, or make real your dreams of romance etc may be true to some extent but it may also be a pipedream that could set you back once reality hits. As I said earlier, addressing underlying issues enough, before you start, is fundamental to maintaining any success later on.

Above hopefully noted....ask yourself and write down:

Why do I want to lose weight?

-

-

-

-

-

-

-

-

-

-

What will being slimmer, achieving a healthier weight, give me that I don't already have..?

-

-

-

-

-

-

-

-

Your list that can be as long as you like but because this is so important we'll be returning to it quite a few times, to keep fine tuning!

Of course how you would like to look, the clothes you'd like to wear, your physical and emotional health may all seem obvious answers.

But take a few moments, maybe even close your eyes, and imagine the person you might be, in three or six months time. Know that these are things you *can* actually make happen, make real for yourself...

Notice what you are wearing:
The colour of your clothes; the texture; the style; the fit...
What are your shoes like?
Notice your hair, whether it is any different.
Notice your posture, how you are standing, or sitting: Weight loss not only alters our appearance when that hunch or roundness has gone from wherever we carry it, it also means we feel different, lighter in spirit, in ourselves, and that will often alter our bearing. It also has a profound effect on the many things that most of us take for granted:
If you are sitting, can you cross your legs?
If you are standing, do you feel somehow taller, more upright?
Can you bend down and touch your toes?
If you are moving around, are you more agile?

Do you have more energy? How do you know?

Can you get up the stairs more easily, even run?

Can you breathe more easily?

Can you sleep better at night?

If you can move around more easily than before and have more energy, do you see yourself joining in more, doing more with friends or partners, children?

How do you feel about being able to join in more?

What would it mean to you?

What would you like to do more of?

How important is it that you can do different things, or appear differently?

-

-

-

-

-

-

Notice whether what you want is measurable, tangible, visible. For example clothes sizes, the scale measurements, what you can fit into and whether you can confidently sit in certain chairs, not need an extension seat belt on the plane, whether you can bend down easily or run very far, if at all. Noticing the ease with which you breathe, sleep, walk.

All of these are things you can see and know.

-

-

-

-

-

-

If your *appearance* is the most important thing for you, how often, where and when will it make the most difference? Whether it's having a far wider choice of off the peg clothes, whether it's out in the wide world or in the intimacy of your bedroom, how badly do you want this?

-

-

-

-

On the other hand there are things which bring quality and happiness into our lives. You might want to feel more *confident,* to have more self worth. But if you include these, make sure you consider how someone else might know you were more confident, energetic, happier etc. What would it look like? What would you be doing? Would you go out more? Accept more invitations? Have a better social life? Would you feel more able to voice your opinion, or stand up for yourself? Might you go for that new job or relationship? Would you feel better able to leave a relationship or workplace that no longer serves you? Would you feel more able to enjoy a relationship you already have?

-

-

-

-

If you believe being slimmer will make you *happier,* ask yourself – how will that show? In what way will I be happier?
Might you smile and laugh more? Be more receptive to others without having to worry about how you feel, or how you believe you're being seen?

-

-

-

Might you simply feel *free* at last? Free from battling, free from self reproach, free from self consciousness, even free from your relationship with food being quite such an issue? Freedom to be you.

-

-

-

-

-

Are you hoping to improve your *health?*

Generally, or specifically?

How important is this to you, how essential is it in terms of life expectancy?

Is there a family history of weight related disease which would be greatly reduced with a healthier weight and healthier eating patterns?

Do you need to drastically reduce blood pressure? Cholesterol levels?

Are you hoping to avoid statins if the cholesterol can be kept down?

Are you hoping to avoid type 2 diabetes, frequently weight related, and accompanying medications?

Are you hoping to be able to conceive, and be healthier while pregnant?

Do you need to lose weight to begin IVF or to have an operation?

Are your joints, knees etc. in danger of damage because of the extra weight?

Has the extra weight brought on asthma, or night time snoring which could be alleviated?

Are you in constant pain that could be helped by being lighter?

Do you have severe reflux which can be helped with reduced eating?

-

-

-

-

For many people, if they feel their weight has really made them stand out, for all the wrong reasons, blending in with the crowd, *feeling normal,* feeling acceptable is absolutely key to their wellbeing.

Is this your motive for losing weight? To feel normal, to fit in, or blend in with the crowd? How important is this to you?

How and where and with whom might you feel this way?

-

-

-

-

-

-

Are you hoping to "*get your life back*"?

If so, what does that mean?

How would your life be different?

Do you believe your life would your life be 10%, 25%, 50% or 100% different?

How do you believe you would feel, and be, compared to now?

-

-

-

-

-

-

If your reasons are general, get as specific as you can. The more vivid the picture, or the feel of what you are wanting, again, the more likely it will impact that part of you that forgets and goes into override, again and again. The idea is that when impulse strikes, you'll at least remember why you're trying to hold back and get one over on the habit of eating for a throw away reason.

Notice too what really pulls or has a strong emotional affect when you think of it. Go through your list and grade your feelings or thoughts up to 10 for the most intense. What is the feeling? How powerful is that feeling or thought? What is the thought? Does it affect you physically in any way? If so, where in your body are you conscious of it?

-

-

-

-

The information that our feelings and physical responses give us is often far more reliable than any rationale. We can't pretend it away and it gives a far greater clue as to what really troubles us, drives us.

Ask yourself whether you feel you ought to be losing weight, whether it's more of a should than a desire, and what actually presses your buttons or pulls the heart strings. Doing something because we feel we ought, and assuming there is choice, (as opposed to a red traffic light) often has far less leverage and holding power in terms of motivation than something which our heart bids: using the 1% rule, it's far easier to outwit the desire for instant gratification with another, more deeply felt desire, than something our head tells us.

Whenever there is feeling, there is energy in it. That energy is the fuel to get us started and carry us through and then keep us there.

Go back to your list again and this time, put them in order of emotional value. Remember we're looking for strength and intensity of feeling here, as opposed to just rationale. Rationale may get you past the first doughnut, but not the second, etc...

-

-

-

-

Now choose your top three, or four or five!

-

-

-

-

Rate how much you want them and how important they are to you, from 1 to 10.

-

-

-

-

It doesn't matter whether your top choices are serious or seemingly trivial. Again it's not about "should" or "ought" but where the feeling is strongest.

If your deepest desire is to strut the beach in your tiniest bikini or speedos, you run with that. You can get help later for the speedos!

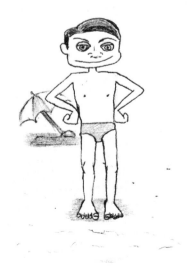

One of the main questions is always **do I want this enough** to steer me through temptation, enough of the time?

Is the thought of whatever tops my list enough to override temptation, **enough** of the time?

To help, imagine you already have whatever it is you most long for. Imagine you have woken up one morning, the weight is off, (and of course your eating patterns have moderated!) and you are free! How do you feel? Ecstatic? Grateful? Relieved? Different?

It's worth mentioning that if you feel **no** different, or sceptical even, this will be relevant and needs checking out: whether you doubt yourself or it simply after all isn't such an issue for you, the check list on pay offs for staying as you are in the chapter on Levels of Motivation, may offer insight.

Ask yourself how will it be a year from now if you achieve this and hold onto it?

How will it be a year from now if you don't? How disappointed or upset might you be?

-

-

-

-

How *clear* is your picture?

By now you'll be getting not just a clearer picture of what it is you want but hopefully a more accurate one. You're going to have a better idea of what it really means to you and what's at stake.

The more vivid that picture gets, the more indelibly it'll imprint itself into the part of you that needs to overcome temptation later on. It's your "As if" image which includes in one template everything that being slimmer holds for you. You might think you'll never forget and never screw up what you've worked so hard to achieve, but something about our behaviour when we're tired and push comes to shove is akin to having a monkey in the driving seat.

Anyone who's been a yo-yo dieter knows this, and even more poignantly anyone who's achieved a normal weight then returned slowly but surely back up to morbid obesity.

What you want eventually is an internal image that you can call upon at will. Becoming able to exert your will over the impulse of the moment, when you choose, creates powerful psychological muscle which will serve you time and again. It is *the* highest act of inner authority. One client was ecstatic when she'd popped into a newsagent to get a bottle of water and not realised until arriving home that she'd "forgotten" to get any of the old treats. High on her agenda had been freedom from constant preoccupation with food and eating. It not even being an issue. She described her forgetting as "the bridge to the road to nirvana!"

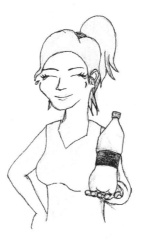

"...the bridge to the road to Nirvana...."[5]

If your top item at the least doesn't have some of this effect, and assuming you are not "doing" denial or that something else in your life doesn't hold far greater priority at the moment, you either haven't quite hit the spot, or it's simply not important enough to you. And by the way that really is *ok*... You can't force motivation or a way of being, and if it isn't there you simply may not have the energy at this present time to take you through

[5] Nirvana: In Bhuddist philosophy it refers the the" stillness of the mind after the fires of desire have been extinguished." Hence the relief!

and beyond. You can't push the river. Realising this will save you a lot of time and effort, not to mention utter angst at putting all the weight back on again because you weren't honest with yourself in the first place and didn't have the necessary drive... which may re-emerge at a later time.

Line of sight...
Once you have your list it's an idea to pin it up somewhere you can see it and add to whenever you need. For a lot of people now that's their iphone but equally having hard copy somewhere your line of sight falls upon, even peripherally day or night, is more likely to keep it alive and filter into your less conscious thoughts and behaviour. Since habits pop up unbidden from the subconscious recesses of our minds, the more a clear quality of intent filters through into these areas, the more chance we have of harnessing impulse and habits in the long run.

When you're done, **date** it.

Anchor it in.
Once a day, for a few moments, wherever you are, bring to mind the image and with a deep inhalation take it down to your solar plexus or tummy. This is your power centre. Breathing normally but softly, hold it there for thirty seconds or so, before letting it go. Over the weeks this will become an anchor point you can call up at will. It will help you override the bit of you that tends to forget when old habits emerge. It will strengthen your resolve and bring back focus.

Remember to focus on the positive, on what you most want:
It is very, very easy to keep slipping back to where we believe we have failed when what you need is the opposite: as with any new venture, anticipation and excitement take us a long way – and it's exactly that energy we want to tap into and hold within us. Hopefully as with my story below, it might happen naturally, but if not, you do need to practise. Just a minute or two every day even, but it does need nurturing!

* * *

The power of the picture:

Just as an example on the value of keeping focus and keeping your eye on the prize… a year or so after I'd left my parental home I was so horribly poor that once a week I'd cheer myself up by going to the Oxford Street travel agency over the road from where I worked in London. I'd pore through the glossy brochures, and then with great care I'd choose one to take away, on the pretext of taking time to consider. I have no doubt the people who worked there must have thought I had a screw loose, especially as I maintained this ritual over the months. About once a day in the office I'd pull the latest one from the top of the growing pile in the drawer, and take equal care and great deliberation choosing my favourite resort. When outside of tea breaks I could hardly be witnessed indulging this habit and wasting office time, I'd find myself daydreaming and bringing to mind the mental image of that week's choice with sublime ease.

Within a year I changed from being an ad rep to long haul cabin crew with BOAC, and over the first 12 months with the airline I ended up at *every single* place I had chosen during my time at that office. I know because I ticked them off, one by one. Whether this is extraordinary testimony to the miracle of manifestation, I will never fully know, though I have pulled off this trick a few times in my life, but what it does highlight magnificently is the power of bringing to mind a mental image, especially when that mental image is vibrant with feeling. Ditto the Bridget Jones type reverie, where it actually becomes a feat of willpower to **stop** the image or thoughts of a new romance wandering into one's work time space…!! The point is that that's the quality of sharpness you are aiming at with your picture. It's got to feel so compelling that every time we're about to succumb to something unnecessary, however appealing in the moment, we are able to ride on by. The more you have a vivid image of both your newfound slimness together with its amazing "benefits package," the more successful you'll be at sidestepping pitfalls.

Motivation is the fuel…

GOAL SETTING AND SETTING YOUR INTENTION

GOAL SETTING:

What *is* your first goal? How clear is your time frame?
By now you will have a clear idea of how ***ready*** you are, and what it is you actually ***want.*** Or you may know what you want, but feel uncertain about other areas of your life being settled enough to enable the focus you need to at least get started and under way.

Your *first* goal:
Often the first "goal" is in fact less about the weight but more about paying attention to issues which repeatedly take you off track. As you read through the Social and Emotional spectrums some of these may become obvious, and addressing these as much as you are able *is* part of the goal. As I said at the outset, the diet part is simply one piece of the jigsaw. If your success with dieting has been temporary, at best, then working with the areas which somehow sabotage your best efforts *is* a vital part of the equation.

Might there be an under-riding belief that you will fail, or some other consequence of your revising your eating behaviours? If you are unsure, Reasons ***not*** to Lose Weight, or Pay Offs for staying as you are - in the chapter on Motivation - will help clarify. However strong your desire to lose weight or maintain what you have lost, if there is a powerful reason to the contrary undermining your best efforts, this absolutely has to be looked at first. It doesn't mean you have to fully resolve something but if that something keeps knocking you off your stride, it will need some degree of attention. Occasionally simply noticing will do the trick. Other times it's far more complex:

Some years ago one of my clients had lost over eight stone, twice, (elsewhere I hasten to add!) when she came to me for a third attempt. This time Jenny disclosed not only that she and her husband had not been intimate for over ten years, but that he had neither touched nor spoken to her directly for nigh on five years, using the teenage children as intermediaries to communicate. Clearly heartbreaking, but a critical time in their schooling as well as finances, the usual, made any kind of moving on seemingly impossible, and although Jenny was a highly practical and upbeat person, she was understandably totally drained and demoralised by her isolation. Compounded by other complexities and including her choice of non disclosure with anyone whose sharing might have afforded some small comfort, her use of food had become an all consuming compensation.

Discussing this with her it was clear that until Jenny could address some of her continuing situation, even by virtue of her emotional reaction to it, there would be little point in losing the weight for the same bounce back to happen yet again.

In this instance while damage limitation and holding her current weight from spiralling further was a main objective, it was none the less secondary to her addressing her now intolerable situation. Even by virtue of discussing it openly for the first time, as well as being able to set a time frame with some kind of end in sight, this was her primary goal for the time being. For the record, Jenny began her weight loss as her children left home to go to university, and last I heard, she had divorced and kept most of it off for some years.

Of course this is an extreme example, but hopefully makes the point. Becoming as *specific* as you are able with regards to ensuring you are readier than you have ever been before in whatever way is pertinent to you, really *is* your initial goal.

Your time frame:
A goal without a time frame is simply a wish. It might happen, but it might not. Further, it comes with an escape clause as we haven't "set ourselves up" for either failure or success. To be sure your intent is indeed a *settled decision* and that it's going to actually happen, there needs to be a way of battening down the hatches, and over and above a revised approach, setting a parameter of time does that job.

Make it *achievable*:

Proof of this is that "actually starting and setting milestones" often elicits anything from a heightened anticipation, to apprehension and fear. Should negative feelings such as fear become debilitating, you might want to check first whether anything else needs sorting by way of preparation, as already discussed, or it might be that you need to take small steps, and go day by day, or week by week. It really doesn't matter how small the steps are, providing, Montessori style[6], they are meaningful and above all achievable. Again, a preliminary goal for many people might even be getting past a previously unattainable first or second milestone.

Word to the wise:

I have frequently heard people remonstrate, as if throwing down the gauntlet to a dieting offender, that a slow, sensible, conventional diet, or eating plan, is the best way to lose weight. Well of course it is! This is categorically one hundred per cent true! Clearly if whatever we change by way of food content or quantity is small but sustainable, you're onto a winner and that is the way to go. The problem for many over consumers is that the minimal reward of a pound loss per week stretches one's ability for delayed gratification to the absolute limit. Not to mention the speed with which one lapse undoes the good work... Many of us, and I include myself here, need enough of a "weight loss reward" in the first few weeks to offset the loss of the "eating reward." It may also depend however on *why* and how come you put on the weight in the first place: if, other than a now resolved situation precipitating the increased eating, or an injury which is now healed, your eating patterns are historically disciplined, the slow conventional pound a week will do just fine.

If conversely your eating behaviours have been reward based or compensating, you may need a faster rate of loss at least until you are sufficiently under way. Again – knowing yourself, and how you operate, is pivotal.

---

[6] Dr Maria Montessori (1870 – 1952) Founder of the Montessori method of education

Whatever you choose however, must again be *specific:* "I'll see how it goes" is more often than not a recipe for disaster and not fit for purpose. To this end, take heed of a widely accepted acronym for goal attainment:

S: Specific
M: Measurable
A: Achievable
R: Realistic
T: Timed

I once had an eyebrow raised by the brilliantly engaging Deanne Jade, founder of The National Centre for Eating Disorders[7], when I confessed that I weigh myself every morning. I understood this daily monitoring to run counter to her concept of best weight management practice implying, possibly, an underlying question about myself. Despite reflection over the years this still rather eludes me though I believe she is correct. Perhaps like Piglet in Winnie the Pooh, (an unwittingly apt choice of character…) I need to be "certain of myself." Of greater relevance however, is her describing herself as having had "a passing experience with anorexia", whilst I, having briefly reached the 3 stone mark a couple of times, would describe myself as having had the opposite, be it equally transitional experience with obesity. The point is that as such we come from different ends of the equation and more pertinently, what I do *works* for *me*: my weight is stable enough; I am healthy; if I put weight on, I do not go into a reactive state of apoplexy and overeating but redress it as and when it occurs, for the most part. In other words, I *respond* rather than react, and I respond appropriately and effectively. What is important is what works for *you.*

So if you have eating and hence weight issues, most people will do well to get themselves weighing scales, which do not need to be expensive so long as they are accurate. But the clue to whether you should weigh yourself once a day or once a week or once a month is really down to your

---

[7] Deanne Jade – Founder and Principal of the National Centre for Eating Disorders (NCFED)

reaction as well as whatever keeps you contained as it were, with your eye on the ball. For me knowing I have put on 2lbs or more after a heavy weekend means I take action with immediate effect. If you wait till the clothes feel tight, you may already be 5lbs plus, and are (possibly) more likely to elicit the knee jerk reaction that serves only to make most of us eat more. You don't want the knee jerk reaction any more than you want denial!

⬅——————————————————————➡

knee jerk reaction　　　　*weighing often enough*　　　　*denial*
　　　　　　　　　　　　　regularly enough for
　　　　　　　　　　　　　　　you!

There are of course other ways to measure, including the use of a tape for chest, waist and hips, and dress or clothes size. I would suggest this on a weekly or monthly basis anyway, although be aware that other factors such as time of the month for ladies, and heat, or even illness can cause fluid retention and alter the figures. Altitude also significantly affects this and when I worked as cabin crew all the women had two buttons an inch apart for comfort while working, to the extent that I could often not get into my smaller jeans and skirts till a couple of days after landing. So be warned, never never weigh yourselves directly after getting off a flight, or for that matter, in the evenings!! The morning weigh in is the one that is least variable, and hence the most reliable!!

The above are all visible but in addition might be the re-emergence of physical or psychological factors that had dropped off as you previously lost weight - which is one of the reasons for keeping a list of even the smallest changes on the way down the scales: Often someone whose renewed sense of self worth meant they were once more going out and socializing, might go back into their shell, or find excuses to stay at home. Or you could find body gestures returning such as arms folded or shoulders slumped, and a general despondency affecting your posture and how you walk. Conversely your energy might once again plummet or your breathing become more strained. Any of these may sound the alarm if you have stopped using scales to check your weight. The subtlety however, could undermine the need for your eyes to be opened, fast, so these are best not relied upon as the sole method for conscious weight holding!

Make it measurable: get those scales!!

Setting your Intention: LETTER to YOURSELF!!

When I am working I interweave constantly between the practical and the psychological, and because many of our habits are so firmly rooted in the unconscious – I will go down every which way to access the automatic behaviours operating from behind the scenes. Similarly, when thinking about your eating habits and the changes you intend to make, it is useful to appeal not merely to your rational mind but to the feeling part of you, as that's the bit that tends to attach itself to your desire to fill a gap with eating either the wrong foods, or more than you need, or drinking or smoking etc.

So to come in from yet another angle and enhance your best possible outcome, I'd like you to imagine you are writing a letter for someone incredibly special in your life. It could be a child, a partner, a parent, or a dear friend whose heartfelt desires are your own and whose happiness you cherish. What you tap into is that wonderful feel good factor which takes us to the best we can be: the kind of feeling that Scrooge might have had after his epiphany in "A Christmas Carol" as he threw open his windows and wished everyone a happy and wonderful day, or the increasing delight of the young Trevor in the film "Pay it Forward" as inspired by his teacher he sets in motion the act of repaying good deeds, not back, but forward ...

The incredibly special person however, will be you. If you find it easier, imagine yourself as a child, or a younger person. As you write your letter, include everything you would hope for yourself and intend to make real by becoming healthier, lighter, becoming free from a controlling habit and whatever was top priority on your list for getting slimmer. Go to town with this and envisage the delight of that younger person as they are so perfectly supported with your gift of love and positive intent.

If you feel drawn to add to your letter at any time, do so.

If it creates a feeling of warmth that you may not have experienced toward yourself for a long time, tap into that whenever you can. This is not about indulgence but rather the healing and happiness that derives from honouring ourselves, acknowledging our foremost needs and keeping to our intent.

Sometimes it's fun to post it, as receiving and opening what we have written to ourselves adds the seal of authenticity!

When you're done, sign it, date it, and put it somewhere you can see.

Dear ....

....

....

....

....

....

....

....

....

....

....

....

....

....

....

LETTER to my BODY:

On a similar basis, and for the same reasons, you can write a letter to your body:

Many people feel loathing for a body that has become overweight and tired; they speak disparagingly and abuse it further by stuffing even more food in or getting angry when "it" doesn't lose the weight fast enough…

In this letter to your body, reflect on the many ways it has served you.

How has your body enabled you to be active?

How has your body felt when you have kept it fit?

How has your body connected you with others?

In love? In motherhood, fatherhood? In dance, in song?

Let your body know how much you appreciate it and value all it has given you. Be specific. Allow it to be heartfelt.

How can you most ensure your body is valued as it deserves?

Let your body know how you will best look after it and treat it with the sacredness it deserves.

Sign and date it. Put it somewhere you will see.

Dear Body.............................

BEST WEIGHT SAFETY NET and...
BECOMING A SKILLED WEIGHT *HOLDER:*

On the basis that "I've blown it!" sets off many a road back up the scales, I am including the **best weight safety net** both here, as well as in Tricks of the Trade, later on.

Assuming you attain a weight or clothes size you're happy with, keeping it steady and becoming a Skilled Weight *Holder,* will be paramount.

Many dieters have a particular weight in mind but give either too much or too little leeway for movement, which is a bit like trying to balance on a five penny piece. Worse, any minor escalation up the scales is either ignored or met with adverse reaction and the rest is history. There are many variations on the trail back up, but key to keeping your weight in balance is to factor in a window for movement which acts as a safety net. It starts to internalise a braking mechanism at a lower point than before. Both in terms of your weight *and* the adverse reaction. However many calories might have been imbibed to incur a slight increase, it's more usually a person's take on it which exacerbates the old eating behaviours and a return to old habits. The safety net helps keep that at bay. Of greater note is that many people who successfully manage their weight have factored this in almost intuitively.

Thinking like a slim person: WINDOW for MOVEMENT
Whatever weight you are aiming to hold, even if you are planning to lose more at a later stage, pinpointing incremental stages of weight gain and what action you might take at each stage will help keep you alert. This does *not* include fluid retention whether hormonal or because you've been on a long flight... and these must be allowed for. Fluid retention is not weight gain. It's called being human, or most of the time, being female! Allow for it!

72

POSITION ONE REFERENCE POINT:

Anyone who has been very overweight or obese for a long time may find it difficult to know what is right for them and have no secure reference point. Wherever you are on the scales, if you intend to hold that weight for any length of time, use *that* for the time being as your guide.

I will refer to this as **Position One**, and going *back* to this as **Return to Base**!

The more you are able to do this when you need, without the "I've blown it" factor coming back in, the more you are getting the knack of becoming a **highly skilled weight holder!**

People who over indulge but seem to manage their eating behaviours enough of the time, (the 1% factor) *do this enough of the time.*

It stands to reason that **Returning to Base** say after a 2 to 3 or 4lb "**oops**" is always best practice. It's less reactive, it's quick to achieve, and succeeding puts us back into a very positive mindset.

I tend to have four stages, but you can create your own.

Stage One:	**Oops!**	2 to 3lbs above original weight
Stage Two:	**Cause for Concern!**	4 to 5lbs above original weight
Stage Three:	**Extra Cause for Concern!**	5 to 7lbs above original weight
Stage Four:	**All Systems Alert!! Houston, we have a Problem!**	8 to 10lbs above original weight or going into the next milestone

OOPs! 2 to 3lbs:

There's a big difference between yo-yo dieting and the slight oscillation which involves an increasingly disciplined Return to Base.

The better you get at doing this within a 2 to 3lb mark, the more automatic it will become. Better still, the new habit will begin to pre-empt any negative thinking which used to get in the way – and allow you scope for a good weekend! What we'll be looking at throughout the book is upping the awareness so you can sidestep the old patterns before they suck you back in!

CAUSE (or extra cause) **for CONCERN**: 4 to 5lbs and 5 to 7lbs:
So you've had a run of great nights out, Christmas, religious festivals, birthdays, whatever, or you've slipped back into your old ways: if you've ignored the first few pounds or simply not managed to take stock, do so NOW!! If you pass the half stone mark, it isn't so much the weight that's a problem as the thinking and feelings that start to go with it. "I've blown it" and other modes of despondency are highly fattening thought processes which make them the road to ruin.
Return to Base with Immediate Effect!

HOUSTON – We have a problem!! All systems ALERT!! - 8 to 10lbs plus…
Both noticing others and in my own experience, the fascinating thing, if you can still *be* fascinated in a kind of macabre way at your own demise by this stage, is the emergence of a particularly negative thought strain. With the toxicity of a computer virus and bent on self destruct, it's a brain change with legs and a force field of its own.

As I say, fascinating, compelling in the extreme, and a great example of the pull of the unconscious. Or automatic pilot – in serious action.

You do not want to go there!

Especially if the 8lb mark is taking you up into the next stone, do everything in your power to **turn back** before this stage. Do not delude yourself that you'll get it sorted at some later point. There's something about a fresh new stone that seems to offer a perverse sense of extra mileage to whatever part of our brain has now taken over! The further you go, the harder it gets to pull back the tide.

Prioritize Returning to Base as if your emotional wellbeing and health were at stake. They may be.

Your WAKE UP CALLS!!

I appreciate this may all sound vaguely alarmist. Maybe leave out the vaguely. But after years in the field, I'd flag up two main areas for real concern: One is addiction, when despite doing everything possible, there is a physical and emotional pull toward eating which is over and above and needs a deeper level of help and support.

The other, at its simplest, is lack of sufficient recognition. When we could have got things sorted at an earlier stage but kept putting it on the back burner. Assuming we are able, that we do have choice and that no other priorities take precedence at a particular point, then yes, this is a **wake up call to action now!** Later will always be harder, with areas of your life ending up on hold.

Hence the mad hand and flag waving, jumping up and down from this end. John Cleese in Fawlty Towers style. I like to work with humour but I hope I have your attention! Take heed!!

Don't make a milestone your millstone!

KEEPING VIGIL!

Earlier I suggested making a list in addition to weighing:

When we start any project of our own choosing, our motivation is usually quite high.

When it concerns our eating behaviours and accumulated weight, it often comes with a level of desperation, which is also quite high.

The problem when we focus on the weight alone is that as we achieve our target the desperation understandably lessens, along with the initial level of motivation. Worse, complacency, a common enough feature of our ability to adapt, enters left of field and we begin to forget or assume we have things sorted and underestimate the combined power of temptation and circumstance. Next we know, the weight has begun creeping and so the struggle begins anew.

Brand new start:

Desperation high...   *Motivation high...*   *Weight high...*

——➤

As time goes by:

Weight goes down...   *Desperation goes*   *But so does the*
                              down...   *motivation...*

At risk of the rhyme sounding like rap, (another idea to keep alert...!) one way of maintaining motivation is for your **appreciation** to stay high. The appreciation however, is not just about the weight and how you look but the many many plusses it brings with it.

MAKE A LIST:

So, from when you begin the new, possibly moderated eating regime, notice *anything* on a daily basis which is a beneficial spin off. Add it to your list. As the list grows, it has several effects:

1. The fact of your *doing* it maintains awareness and an alertness. It isn't about obsessing. It's like any new field of study or job we keep focus till we can do it without thinking, as with learning to drive.

2. The fact of doing it is testimony to your commitment. It shows you are serious.

3. As the list grows you will appreciate increasingly that it is as much about a **quality of life** that often has an invaluable benefits package. **That's** the bit you are far less likely to turn a blind eye to if you find old habits returning.

4. As and when weight starts to creep... should you go into any kind of denial, it's not so easy to ignore the list as it makes a u-turn.

YOUR LIST!!
(Have a few gold stars at the ready! You're worth it and it draws the attention!!)

-
-
-
-
-
-
-
-
-
-
-
-
-
-
-
-
-
-
-

yes it should be a long list......!

-
-
-
-

LEVELS OF MOTIVATION
AND
MOTIVATION OVER TIME:
YOUR MoT

LEVELS of MOTIVATION:

In "What gets in the Way" I mentioned one of the predominant pitfalls being a lack of factoring in the varying levels of motivation. Because it features so strongly I go into some depth to highlight what goes on:

The three main levels:

Emergency motivation;

Reward based motivation;

Long term motivation;

People beat themselves with the lack of willpower stick, but it's pretty difficult to keep a tight grip on something, all of the time. And when our level of resolve weakens, be it, by the degree, by an almost inaudible heartbeat, it isn't always that we want that something any less, but that there are varying stages of motivation.

Emergency Motivation: first level...
Emergency Motivation can be life saving and in line with our fight or flight survival mechanism, it isn't designed to continue. It's the psychological equivalent of the adrenalin which enables us to almost superhuman strength in emergencies: the parent who lifts a car to free a trapped child; the soldier who runs carrying his wounded mate. More benignly the extraordinary surge of strength which enabled a wearying Mo Farah to win back the lead apparently against all odds in the 10,000 metre race at the London 2012 Olympics! If you watched it, wasn't that something!!

With this kind of motivation it's back against the wall, desperation crisis, do or die. We can no longer see a way out, other than doing the thing we have long put off, feared we'd fail at, or didn't have the juice for. But now urgency or passion has created that juice and something else is at stake, like our health, our self esteem, our sanity, a job, a relationship, some situation, whatever, has upped the ante. This is ***rocket fuel*** in terms of getting launched. The trick with this level of motivation is that once that rocket is launched and you are – sweet mother of mercy on your way, do not assume this state of heightened focus will continue should you take a short break because it isn't meant to: carry on until your trousers are dropping off from the reduced waist band or the measurement on the scales is reading a healthy place to be. Because if you stop for ANY other reason, the Desperation Juice is rarely there in such potent form when you try to pick up from where you were before. You have moved away from Emergency Level and the launching fuel has lost its punch. You're no longer firing on all cylinders or bouncing off the same diving board.

Reward Based Motivation: second level...

There's still a way to go but the excitement of the results on a weekly basis continue to reward you for all the effort put in, as well as the reward at the end, and is enough to keep you going... most of the time. It's a challenge, but there is still resolve. Again, even more than before, do not look back, do not look down. Eyes forward, focus on the prize. Dithering, or worse, rewarding yourself for "being so good" with the hair of the dog that took you up this merry path in the first place, is as crazy as a heroin addict relenting on cold turkey three days in. Ok, this is mostly pertinent to those of you whose health and wellbeing is seriously jeopardised with the weight you are carrying. I know a lot gets blamed on weight, (infuriating at times...) but if the correlation between your knee joints being shot to pieces and your weight soaring sky high is overwhelming, clearly, this applies. A lot of your friends are going, yeah, go on go on, treat yourself, while anyone who half way gets this scenario would be crying out No!! Begging you "Don't do it!!", "Hold your ground!", "Only a while to go!!" Granted, I sound just a little demented, but I've seen the slow incline back *up* the scales, way too many times. And yes, of course no one can believe at the outset that anyone in their right mind would remotely risk ruining all the hard work. But this *is* the thing about "unconscious behaviour" or the "automatic impulse". It happens when that other you, the one who is not of so sound mind because of the many reasons we'll be looking and exploring, is suddenly in charge. It's like there's a lunatic at the head of the train. Recognizing how and when we get like that is part of the way forward. Take heed!!

Long term Motivation or Motivation over Time (MoT): third level...
Long term or Motivation over Time is the one that people stop at for a short while and then, judging by statistics... lose sight of after 6 to 12 months and slippedy-slide all the way back up again. This is the point at which we seem to become the most complacent or unconscious, yet actually requires a greater level of vigilance, of mindfulness, because we are NOT getting an extra reward at the end of each week... or it isn't as noticeable. We already ***have*** the reward, i.e. our slimmer, healthier self, but once we've had it a while it is the easiest thing in the world for it to fade into the background of our daily lives. We park it to the side and no longer give it its sacred due. We have acclimatized to its amazing effects and no longer keep vigil. And that's where things go horribly wrong. If it were a motorway, it would be a notorious accident spot.

The bulk of this book is to enable ***recognition*** of the slow slip back into old patterns, to recognize how and where and when it occurs, and to provide strategies as well as insight to hold new eating behaviours in place. And this... requires long term motivation...

Recognising that if something is important enough you will have to keep incentives in place to carry you through, to ensure there's enough fuel in the energy bucket, is possibly the most significant thing we can get to know about ourselves. This ***is*** part and parcel of the ***motivation mileage test.*** Your ***MoT*** is what you might do to keep the Motivation over Time, in place.

Long term motivation is sustained with four main ingredients:

The first is ***Recognition.*** Usually someone who has fallen foul more than once is more likely to get this. Without sufficient recognition, how can you possibly realise in time when you are treading the same old path, again? It doesn't usually come with a built in alarm system, (though one of the strategies is to do just this...). More likely an imperceptible one off event, rather like a train with just an ever so tiny derailment going off piste by a degree, followed by another and so on.

In line with the above, people often feel their needs are secondary, not weighing up the knock on effect to their lives. Women and mums especially will protest that time taken to focus on themselves is selfish, completely negating the extent to which a happy, smiling, more active way of being impacts positively on the lives of those around them.

Certainly where health is concerned, our capacity to succumb to temptation and override our better judgement even when well informed, is plain to see. Proof that the only leverage that counts when we're trying to give up an enduring habit is indeed, motivation. Recognising this and the importance the outcome holds for you will help you decide *ahead of the game* whether you want to make the effort, or to know that you have to.

The meaning we give consciously or unconsciously to what we're doing, has an immediate knock on effect on our ability to get started, carry on without floundering, and maintain what we've worked so hard to achieve.

The value we afford to our desire to lose weight, maintain that weight, and shift our relationship with food and drink is absolutely in line with the level of priority we give it in our daily lives.

The second is *Desire.* You have to want what being lighter, slimmer, healthier will give you at least 1% more than the extra bit in front of you, enough of the time. And that mental picture of what we want, and moreover, want to *keep,* has to always kick back into place whenever we start to get sloppy. Were you to let areas of your professional life, your work, slip, in the same way we let our attention to sufficient weight management slip, would you still *have* a job?!

The third is *Commitment.* Which of course follows a high enough level of Desire and enables the fourth essential ingredient, *Planning and Prioritizing.*

Planning is pivotal. It is proof of your maintained focus and that the motivation is enduring. The question to ask yourself whenever you go off track is not how come I ate so much, but how come I forgot to *plan,* how come I lost my *focus?* This is much more likely to provide the information you need. If, for example you are mind bendingly tired, it is very, very difficult to keep focus, and not to end up comfort eating. Your objective at this point, somehow or other, is to find ways of getting more sleep or a better quality of sleep.

Prioritizing returns in a way to **Recognition**, but this time it is recognizing whenever the priority we gave to our eating plans and weight loss has somehow slid to the bottom of the pile. As such a lot of this happens again at an unconscious level, I will spend time later looking at ways to pin it into place along with the ***Do I still value this enough?*** motivation mileage test!

For the moment though, dipping deeper into the layers of motivation…

ROCKET FUEL FOR LIFT OFF AND SUCCESS!!
THE POWER OF INCENTIVE and shorter term motivation…
When I'm working with people I tend to differentiate long term from short term motivation. Long term, as it would suggest, enables a shift in mindset that is long lasting, with an enduring change in attitude. The driving force behind it will range from powerful to non negotiable. By contrast, an incentive, which often involves a point in time, is short term. It's main problem is that it will pass, with the tidal pull of all our previous habits flooding back in the wake of its anticlimax. Think weddings and brides, public events… a big run up and then flat line… This may sound a bit dramatic, or rain on your parade, but it's best to have your eyes wide open!! Short term incentives need to come with built in alarm systems… which if you're half way serious, you will build in!! Forewarned is forearmed etc…

… rocket off from Houston horse-power…
However… not to be underestimated in its dynamic, rocket off from Houston launch power, incentives provide invaluable, highly effective stepping stones along the way which I often term **Honeymoon Motivation!** It has a lot of the attributes of emergency motivation but without the crisis.

One of my favourite examples was a lady who felt she desperately needed help to get to a better weight which she wasn't managing on her own, but decided after a few weeks she couldn't afford to keep coming. Several years later she returned, and this time I checked at the outset whether she was financially able to see it through. Apparently not, but her ex husband was coming to her daughter's wedding three months hence with his new wife in tow, and no way was a mere overdraft going to stop her looking as fantastic as she possibly could for the occasion. I never saw or heard from her again after our final meeting so have no idea whether she maintained her new weight, but she did look brilliant and more to the point she was brimming with delight and self confidence. Now *that's* incentive!!

Incentive then, is a ***powerful catalyst:*** it reinforces the behaviour we want, the action we need to take, in the right direction.

What incentives do you have coming up?

If you are planning to attempt weight loss in the near future, do you have any event milestones which could help get wind under your sail, fire up your enthusiasm, crank up the get up and start today mojo?

LIST YOUR INCENTIVES and grade out of 10 your level of really wanting the results:

Weddings, parties, rite of passage birthdays, graduations, college reunions, holidays…?

-

-

-

-

-

-

Whatever you do, be honest with yourself about what lights your fire:

In the groups I've run over the years, I've noticed that in the context of someone having to lose weight to reduce already apparent and increasing risks to their health, others will often apologise and look sheepish over what seems frivolous by comparison. But whether your longing is to fit into a particular pair of jeans or to stay alive to see your children marry and have children themselves, whether it's to not be the pudgy mum waiting at the school gates, or to be able to play footie with your son, is irrelevant. What's relevant is the bit that contains the *most* emotional energy. That's your fuel. Vanity might be a shallow reason compared to big life issues, but the leverage of wanting to look the best we can has mighty lift off power!! Use the momentum!

As you make your list, have a think about whether you have generally begun diets in the past because of similar reasons or some other incentive, only to revert once the occasion is over?

How might that be different this time? What might make the difference?

From the list you made earlier, do you have a more deeply felt conviction this time that could help make that difference?

It's also useful to notice whether it's **reward based incentive,** the short term sprint to something we want, or **escape based incentive,** taking us away from the unwanted.

... carrot on a stick... reward based incentive...

When they fall within the wider framework of a more deeply felt, longer lasting motivation, incentives are especially great stepping stones along the way as much as they can be rocket launchers to get you there in the first place. Incentives usually mean you are *acting in advance,* that there's a carrot on a stick which is why they play their part just as effectively when the new weight is achieved: if you have a beach holiday once a year, it is far easier to use the momentum of looking forward to something to get those few pounds down in anticipation of more of you on show, than it is once you return. It's the reward at the end, **pay it forward** variety of weight maintenance which is just so much easier and so much more likely to actually happen. It has leverage, even if you're only galvanized into real action the last two or three weeks! Which is why it is worth purposely building them into your year once you achieve the new you, to make sure you stay that way!

Let's have a closer look at that second one, *escape based incentive...*

FREEDOM FROM...

Because the desire to escape something is invariably driven by a negative emotion such as pain or fear, it is likely that any incentive in this respect is more of a long term motivation.

The fact of its being *escape driven* doesn't make it any less powerful: fear is a great motivator and pain has a sharp way of keeping our focus... but as pain and desperation reduce, so does motivation, so it's always a good idea to rephrase what you *don't* want into a list of what you *do* want. Or couple the two side by side.

────────────────────────────────▶

What do you most want to...   *and this converts to...*
escape from?   *Leave behind?*

-
-
-
-
-
-
-
-
-
-
-
-
-
-

In one way or another, once we have put on a certain amount of weight, it's remarkably easy to put areas of our lives on hold: it might be as mundane as refusing to buy new or nicer underwear till we've "gone back" to our old weight, or putting our social lives on hold so we can start the famous, eternally deferred diet without being tempted astray. Or it might be far more serious. For some people, and taking on board that how you *feel* about your weight is as significant as the weight itself, being anything from overweight to morbidly obese can be akin to a prison sentence.

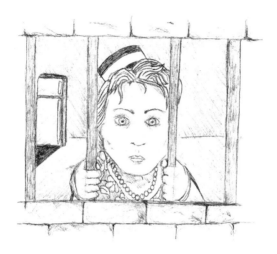

The "WHEN I GET THIN" list:
List how your life is on hold.

Make a list of the things you don't do, or have stopped doing, because of your weight.

-
-
-
-
-
-

What do you find yourself saying you'll do "When I've lost the weight"?

-

-

-

-

-

How long have you been saying that?

-

How else does it restrict you?

-

-

-

-

-

Note down which areas of your life are held back in any way.

-

-

-

-

-

Just to reality check, write down the evidence for this. Be specific.

-

-

-

-

-

Notice how you are affected physically, emotionally, mentally. What are the feelings? Grade their strength with 10 being very strong.

-

-

-

-

-

RED ALERT:
Reiterating here, but to hammer it home. **Reality check** and separate fiction from fact: whilst problems might feel worse and be exacerbated by carrying more weight than is wise, not everything links to your weight. As I said earlier, addressing underlying issues enough, before you start, is fundamental to maintaining any success later on.

OTHER SIDE OF THE COIN:
Reasons not to lose weight: what might stop you?
Might sound mad, but there really are often a set of perks that go with any habit or way of being we've held for a long time, even if it's simply the safety of the familiar. And however valid the reasoning, if you only want to lose weight simply because you feel you ought, or because it's important to someone else, you might continually find yourself lacklustre if not downright resentful about the entire experience. Never mind managing to maintain what you achieve. However beneficial the health improvements, unfortunately the only way this really seems to work and moreover stick, is when you truly want it for yourself.

WEIGHING UP THE PAY OFFS and benefits of staying as you are:
Ask yourself some of the questions below. Notice any immediate top of the head response or gut feeling but allow yourself to reflect on it over time as well and see what comes up for you.

What does being overweight *do* for me?

-

-

Why might I want to stay as I am?

-

-

What are my judgements, or beliefs about other people's judgements?

-

-

What are my fears about having a healthier weight?

-

-

What are the ***pay offs or benefits*** of staying as I am?

-

-

-

-

-

Just in case you're stumped for insight, listed below are some of the reasons people have included over the years which kept them stuck for a while:

- I know inside myself it's going to be a long hard slog and it's a long term commitment. I feel overwhelmed before I even begin.
- If I don't start, I can't fail.
- I don't want to reduce my eating. I don't know if I can.
- It'll ruin my social life if I always have to watch what I eat / drink.

- I feel I might lose my cheerfulness if I become slim, my personality might change.

- I'm worried that being slimmer will make me more attractive and bring temptation from outside of my relationship.

- My partner worries I'll be more attractive and then gets jealous.

- I'm frightened of attracting sexual advances. Being bigger means I get to hide in my body.

- There's hardly any communication or intimacy any more in my relationship and eating is the only sensory enjoyment I have. Actually I can't seem to stop.

- My father / mother always tried to control my weight and said no one would want me / I wouldn't be successful etc. I feel that losing the weight I've put on is like admitting they were right, even though I'm now an adult. Keeping my weight is like asserting my independence still, raising two fingers...

- I love cooking and taking care of people and I might have to restrict some of that to keep my weight down.

- Professional lunches would be awkward if I couldn't eat/drink as much: the clients might feel awkward / I would feel awkward.

- I'm worried my skin will sag when the weight is gone.

- I'm worried I'll look gaunt, unwell or old.

- I feel so feminine the way I am. I don't want to lose that, or my sensuality.

- Being round makes me more like a mummy. More loveable.

- I feel like being big means I hold weight in the world. I know it's not the same but it feels that way.

- Being big means people don't mess with me.

- I feel angry at the world. Being big is like a rebellious act.

- I don't know if I can be different. I'm scared.

- I don't know who I will be under all of this (my weight).

- My life's been on hold for so long because of my weight. Supposing all the things I hope for "when I'm thin," just don't happen? I don't know how I would deal with that, if I could deal with that. There's almost too much at stake.

- Not have to worry about feeling selfish and taking time for myself. It'll be unfair to my children / partner / family...

-

-

-

Whether or not any of these resonate with you, it is really useful to cotton on to anything which could put a dampener on your efforts. If you aren't aware, the effect can be like getting in a car and trying to start while the brakes are still on, then wondering why it's so hard and giving up. Notice whether what you have written feels true to you. Often we swallow assumptions whole and fail to check for any basis in reality, whether there is any *real* evidence to support our belief. Assumptions or beliefs to the contrary can sit unseen below the surface and act as silent saboteurs to our best laid plans. (See later in Distorted Thinking and How We See Things...)

More importantly what comes up for you in the list can highlight issues that need addressing before you even attempt weight loss of any kind.

Apart from the very real and practical realisation of the task ahead, the more emotionally complex reasons for hiding under unnecessary weight, or for extreme emotional eating, simply make a tough journey tougher if you don't really understand what lies beneath. Worse, even if you succeed in achieving a healthy weight, whatever prompted your old eating habits and relationship with food will still be there, pulling you back to where you were before. This doesn't have to mean a total psychological excavation... but a gentle approach to what compels you really is as important as the diet itself.

Deterrents and desperation...

One final look at escape based incentive and emergency motivation...

Possibly one of the most powerful incentives of all other than the do or die wake up call, has to be desperation; when we've meant to do something for so long or felt stuck for so long the torment is no longer bearable, our back is against the wall, and suddenly it's a two way street: despair or survival.

It's amazing what kicks in at beyond the eleventh hour but it's worth remembering that *change can happen fast.* One lady who came to see me tipping the scales at 32 stone reported feeling completely differently about herself within days of changing some of her eating habits. This is not unusual and since such brief time is hardly transformative in weight terms, the transformation is in our perception. Feeling like we're back at the steering wheel and once again in charge of ourselves is crucial to our wellbeing and that is the bit that can happen fast.

Which makes our capacity to revert all the more extraordinary and which puts it in the incentive category, be it a highly motivating one: as I described briefly in Keeping Vigil, this is how it goes – we reach a weight at which we are so deeply unhappy we will now do anything to alleviate the emotional pain we are feeling. Whatever else is going on in our lives that has been more important now takes a place further down the priority scales while sorting ourselves out shifts to the top. Relief and elation the pounds start dropping – initially reinforcing our determination and evangelical fervour as the compliments fly in and the feel good factor soars... and the old dogs of depression and desperation are like dots on a distant horizon. And then something strange happens. Along with the weight going down, and the desperation going down, the motivation goes down as well. It's strange because it's not as if we don't care, because we so do, but it's like once the emergency is over, there's something akin to an adrenalin drop, and the level of resolve which so mercifully kicked in, kicks right out again.

We are of course primed to alleviate the highest given pain at any time, which makes sense, except with humans that includes emotional pain. It's a survival mechanism along with fight or freeze or flight. And if only we could recreate at will that level of resolve without the emergency, what life changing feat of achievement that would be!

Well in fact... that's exactly where we're heading, and on the basis that if you practise anything for long enough, you'll surely improve, this is where the longer lasting motivation comes into its own.

Of course what is happening is that once the pain of desperation subsides, all seems well till the pain of resisting re-emerges. Resisting whatever we feel most deprived of - which is usually whatever lay beneath our overeating or drinking in the first place. Time goes by, and in alleviating that particular pain instead, we succumb to same old same old, the old weight returns and voila, we are back where we started. Sound familiar?

So how do we recreate a level of resolve that will see us through the choppy waters of appetite, desire and habit? Potentially we get to a point, if it is serious enough, (and this varies individually of course,) where the mind numbing waste of time, energy and life itself triggers the buck stops here button. Coupled with the motivation towards what we want instead, something anchors itself into our system, enabling us to put the brakes on much sooner than before, and we are on our way. Whether there is in fact a greater stoicism in the character of those who achieve this, whether they have more to lose or whether they simply "get it" more, who knows. What's exciting is that once you begin to have the edge over where and when and why you overeat, once you get the knack of sidestepping or overriding compulsion... there's a seemingly magical mastery that comes in with the deal and the ripple effect is far reaching...

From where I'm sitting, sidestepping a potential pitfall, whether it's social or emotional – will always be a lot easier than making a choice when you're in it: not buying the dunking doughnut in the first place is a whole lot easier than the effort of restraint once the doughnut is bought.

But we have to remember not to buy the doughnut.

Clearly then, it's as important to have a vivid appreciation of what you no longer want so it's there to deter you every time you're about to fall for a choice that goes in the wrong direction. Like if you bought the doughnut for "someone else" (oh yeah?) and it's been winking at you every time you open the cupboard. As well as keeping their "before" photos on a wall or on the fridge, a lot of people have found it really helpful to have a memory snapshot as it were, of whatever it was made them suddenly go "Hey!! Enough!" A defining **Buck Stops Here** moment in time:

The BUCK STOPS HERE! Moment in time snapshot:
A *buck stops here* snapshot is my term for a deeply felt emotional memory of an experience you'd rather forget. Whether it's a Bridget Jones large underpants moment or something far worse, anchoring it in to your immediately available memory bank will be the shock to the system to remind and help deter you from the old overeating response. Remember, it isn't just the temptation to overeat or drink, it's the *habit* of doing this when we're not even hungry. The habit happens in a heartbeat. So getting to grips with the situations that trigger it and surround it and keep your habit in place is where we're heading. Along with creating a visceral, emotionally, physically felt reminder of what we want and don't want, instead. I labour the point only because habit is such a hard nut to crack unless something very definite can override it.

What is interesting is why some of us are predisposed to reach this moment sooner than others. Almost like a breaking thermostat set to start beeping alarms at a certain weight, for some people that takes far too long. Whether you "do" denial as a way of coping or whether you meet temptation at every turn ... having reminders that can set off keenly felt emotions is rather like setting up flashing lights along a motorway: it's to alert you to danger.

So do you have a particular moment or period of time when something stopped you in your tracks, made you shift gear? Shot the need to make changes right to the top of the **Must do Now!** list?

Make it vivid, make it specific, bring to mind the feelings that came with it. To get the most potent "can't go there ever again / won't go there" effect, the feelings need to go with the image, to be fully visceral. If you felt embarrassment or shame, let yourself feel just enough of it to slot in with the snapshot. It's a slice in time, which will be your personal anti-serum. It will help dislodge the habit from its very secure hidey hole.

One client said she would never forget breaking the seat of a wooden chair as she sat down to watch her little girl in a school play, and worse, finding herself stuck and wedged into it when she attempted to get up later on. No saving grace released her from the sheer indignity of the moment, but it is a "buck stops here" snapshot that has served her well, as you can easily imagine. That is what she brings to mind when she finds herself slipping into old habits.

Cast your mind back and create your own list, but bring it down to the one with the strongest emotional affect. Here are a few that get brought in:

- the holiday photos / video
- the wedding / graduation / party photos or video
- catching yourself in a shop window
- trousers splitting in public
- snotty shop assistant offering a size too big or too small
- caught eating in secret.

Add your own:

-
-
-
-
-
-
-
-
-
-
-

BUCK STOPS HERE MEMORY STICK!

What / when.... was the ACTUAL MOMENT something in you shifted, made a decision? Was it the result of a gradual process, or a defining moment?

-

-

-

-

-

What happened?

-

-

-

-

-

Where is the EMOTIONAL CHARGE, the AFFECT, as you speak or think about it? What are the feelings? Where are they in your body?

-

-

-

-

-

If you're not sure, tell someone your story and you'll know soon enough! Additionally, something in your delivery will soon have their FULL attention. That often holds the emotional charge together with how you'll be feeling...

RED ALERT:

The idea of this is to act as a **motivating deterrent**. An electric shock if you like that goes "No, you so don't want to do that" whenever impulse strikes. Ideally this would happen before rather than after the fact, but we learn with time, and eventually even hindsight becomes foresight. It's designed to be the Pavlov's Dog[8] type of motivation, reinforcing behaviour away from one thing and directing us toward another, except we're setting this up for ourselves. IF however you find it simply distresses and draws you back into destructive eating behaviours, then don't do this. At all times, listen to your own intuition, hear and heed your own inner voice. Many people who overeat have become very skilled at blocking this out. It may be difficult at first to tell the difference between an impulse and what really holds true, but here's the place to begin testing it out.

---

[8] Ivan Pavlov (1849 – 1936) Renowned for his work in Classical Conditioning, he learned of the concept most notably with the "conditioned reflex" of dogs to the buzzer sound which meant food was on its way!

KEEPING TRACK:
EFFECTIVE PRIORITIZING
and
MOTIVATION CHECK

EFFECTIVE PRIORITIZING
And proof of your motivation in action…

There is an infinite assortment of things that we would love, that we believe we need or give importance to, at any time and all the time. We have, as it were, a behind the scenes calculus making choices from the moment we rise and throughout the day that we put into effect with barely a moment's thought: what time we intend to get up, whether we need to leave earlier than usual, whether to have juice or coffee or tea, and so on. Fairly obviously if something is urgent, we give that precedence over everything else. Equally, actions such as cleaning our teeth even when in a massive rush, do not qualify as "urgent" but are routines that most of us would not dream of omitting. So effectively, what we end up doing is the enactment of our prioritizing. There is a kind of value scale going on at any given moment and in order for something to get done, and be kept in the equation rather than deferred or dumped, we have to value it *enough.*

We need this to happen with our eating behaviours and weight maintenance, but the problem is that we often confuse our genuine desire for something with its place on the value scale. I have had a genuine desire to speak impeccable French for thirty years, but my need for that fluency has never quite hit the mark. You appreciate the difference!

Unfortunately our wellbeing is frequently the something that gets relegated low on the priority list: despite the delight and joy that many experience from having achieved a great weight loss, despite its fantastic benefits package as I call it, even though we know it won't just look after itself without a certain level of attention, we somehow forget to pay the piper.

On the basis we tend to vote with our feet, the only reason for allowing something to slip, for continually deferring whatever it takes to lose the weight and then keep that weight off, is either a belief that it needs no further attention and will look after itself, or… that however important it might seem, however much value we believe it holds, the mirror of our actions proves otherwise. And certainly by the second or third time around, the former no longer holds true. So either we are seriously kidding ourselves or... somewhere along the line, the priority we gave to get to this stage, begins to slip. Often it is such a matter of degree that we may not even realise this is the case. Our language, as well as our actions, is often a giveaway in this respect: consider the word "try"...

The *moment* you say you will "*try*" to do something, even supposing you truly believe it is hugely important, the word itself indicates you have already opted for a safety clause which allows for escape or failure. It may seem innocuously nitpicking but imagine by way of example, that you asked a person to pick up 4 year old Johnny or Jane from the school gates at a set time and they said that they would "try": "Trying" would be unacceptable! You'd be horrified! Equally, if you have an important interview, or a job you value, you would always check everything from the alarm clock to the transport to your mobile phone being fully charged to absolutely ensure your arrival on time.

When things start to slip, as a rule at least, somehow and somewhere we relegate it down the priority scale without even being conscious of our doing so. We fail to recognise there is an automatically operating **DO I VALUE THIS ENOUGH** calculus going on in the background which we could then weigh up and factor in. This is about recognising areas which conflict or differ in value strength, often so subtly it is easy to miss, but are crucial and key not merely to goal setting but to keeping what we have already achieved in place. The mirror of our actions says everything and the meaning we give consciously or unconsciously has an immediate knock on effect on our ability to get started, carry on without floundering, and maintain what we've worked so hard to achieve. As I said earlier however, since our focus is more naturally maintained whilst still aiming for the reward of weight loss and all it provides, the period of time most at risk is, as visibly evident with statistics, the in for the long haul weight holding stage.

Effective prioritising is therefore an integral part of long term motivation: the value we afford to our desire to lose weight, maintain that weight and shift our relationship with food and drink is absolutely in line with the level of priority we give it in our daily lives. Of course stuff gets in the way, and by the time you have flagged up what and when and how and why with the social and emotional spectrums, you will be more clued in than ever before. Even the obvious is never obvious enough. But there is a subtle difference between finding creative ways to maintain a better eating plan when circumstances are very challenging, and not appreciating that its value has lost its hold. Often there is an assumption about time needing to be taken in a day already too full, which might only need a few tiny changes to hold things sufficiently in place. But we need to know it's going on.

To put this in perspective - if there were something screwing up your best efforts at work, however mundane, or putting your child's health at risk, you'd leave no stone unturned and would give it your 100% attention. That *quality* of attention, of focus, of Hercule Poirot with monocle and magnifying glass scrutiny – is what works. Attention to detail is paramount though it may not always start with the obvious. A lot of weight gain is as much due to a mountain of the mundane as it might be to deeply complex emotional issues.

Your proof of the pudding 24/7 camera crew!!
So do we value it **enough,** and if we have areas that are stalemating each other, are we even aware of it? Should you not be sure, other than a fluctuating number on your weighing scales, imagine one of those Big Brother national reality programmes with millions of us tuned in to watching your eating behaviours 24/7… (how horrible can it get!). Imagine we have been told you have revised your eating, and are aiming to lose weight, or, to **hold** and maintain your weight where it is. There is however no sound, and no subtitles, so we are not privy to your thoughts.

What would we see?
What would it look like?
Would your actions be testimony to your intentions?!!!
What might we be looking for…?

Once you have read through the social, emotional and physical spectrums, you will have a much better idea of the kind of things that can affect your eating behaviours but by flagging this up now, you can be more on the alert!

If for example, you are someone whose lack of sleep is weakening any resolve to keep comfort foods at bay, your valuing of the need for this would ensure you find ways of getting to bed earlier.

You might make a real point of filling up with petrol early in the day when you are less likely to go for the goodies.

You'd make sure the tempting food items you've bought for the family are hidden at the back of an upper shelf, out of immediate view.

You'd maintain your effort to plan ahead so you're not caught short when out or at work, with too long between meals....

With each of the above, until such actions become **habitual,** you might have to set things up to **remind** you. With time any effort is rewarded as your prioritizing becomes automatic. This not only prevents any unconscious forgetting, it also means there is no longer the drain on energy that comes from conflict: the job is done so there *is* no conflict.

This is again however, where a **reminder** on your wall someplace, along with the internalised image of what you really want, and want to **keep,** comes into its own. This way it will stay as something you remember over and again that you **want,** and doesn't therefore get relegated to the **should** and **ought status** which is brain draining, depleting, and usually guarantees going to the "*forgotten*" pile.

Valuing your weight maintenance enough means you will make the effort to put reminders in place. If you think about the many ways in which we use memory sticks, post it notes, mobile phone alarms, lest we forget something important, and this is often in our highly developed areas, areas of strength, why on earth would we not use this similarly to support our weight maintenance...? Again, whether or not we are conscious of it, it is an authentic indication of our level of valuing. Proof of the pudding!

Alert!! Review!!

If you're becoming increasingly aware of feeling like you should or ought to be doing this and that with regard to maintaining healthy enough eating plans, that could also be one of those *red warning lights!* It's very difficult to make yourself do something which is fast becoming an irritation and is not legally imperative… so if this is the case it's time to review your earlier motivation, and what it is you wanted. You may indeed choose to let things ride, but at least you'll be conscious of it, you'll be sure of why, and the consequences.

COLLECTING the EVIDENCE! *(More detective work…)*
The DO I VALUE IT *ENOUGH* LIST:

By way of setting a reference point for yourself, make a list of everything which you do *daily or weekly or monthly* that could, in essence, be left out, but *isn't.* You therefore make a choice to include it. Think carefully as much of this will include things you take for granted. Your valuing of them is so high, it's a non negotiable. I do *not* include something like getting dressed, unless you never leave the house, as most of us would probably prefer not to shop naked. (Naturists notwithstanding!) I do however include something like cleaning one's teeth once, twice, or three times a day. Your personal hygiene is one of your foremost value systems in action. We assume a norm, yet it is very variable.

You might also include something like checking bank statements, or ironing your underwear. Yes, I actually have a friend who does this (ironing his pants) who was horrified to discover that I do not. Yes, it is a "he", and this takes time in a day which is already crammed full. My assumption, which I must check, is that this is in fact his time for reflection, "allowable" inasmuch that it is productive. If this is the case, it's a great example of his valuing a need, and installing it into his schedule.

Another dear friend who frequently complains he hasn't the time to write as much as he would like, makes time none the less to go running for at least an hour a day. It says everything.

I, by contrast, will make time for writing, but find it "difficult" to "fit in" the amount of activity I would like for my back side not to get rigor mortis over the hours.

Checking for chain reactions...

What we're looking for, in relation to eating patterns, is what seems to make keeping your weight steady more of a challenge, when in fact it's the end result of *personal choice* rather than the inevitable.

For anyone familiar with those swinging metal balls that became a popular desktop feature in the seventies, they might easily evoke a great mental image of the knock on effects between each and every thought, feeling, choice and subsequent actions and eating behaviours. Our overeating is rarely an isolated incident but part of a chain of events.

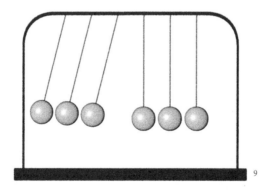

So.... Your List:

Initially all you have to do is to notice.

Ideally, *take* note and write it down or put it on your phone. Sometimes that really is enough. the more we realise how minimal effort reaps great rewards, the less we'll keep putting it off and making it an even bigger deal.

---

[9] Newton's Cradle – (sometimes called the Executive Ball Clicker) – named after Sir Isaac Newton, is a device that demonstrates continuation of momentum and energy via a series of swinging spheres.

Notice whether things you believe have to be done are genuinely imperative, or whether it is in fact your belief, and therefore your choice.

Things you *choose* to do:

-
-
-
-
-
-

Things you believe you *have* to do.

-
-
-
-
-
-
-
-
-

What *needs* to be reinstated?
Now think about what needs to be put into place, or stay in place, that helped you maintain your eating plans before and which have slipped.

Make a list and write down how much time each of these would take.

How much time would they actually take from your day or week?

Remember this might not always be the most obvious. Getting to bed earlier to get enough sleep so that we are less vulnerable to temptation, is one, but equally so is ringing a friend because you feel restored, and that boosts your general resolve. Or it might be drinking enough fluids or taking a longer route to avoid the fast food outlets on your way home. Think laterally as well as practically!

-

-

-

-

-

-

-

-

Finally, what would be the positive effect of making, or reinstating, changes that enabled your steadier weight maintenance?

Remind yourself of all you said you wanted at the beginning. Everything you believe being in charge of your eating behaviours and your weight and health, will give you. Even finding ways to remember to keep that image uppermost in your mind, is proof of your level of valuing.

-

-

-

-

-

-

-

None of this is about right or wrong, it is simply to get clear on the choices we are making, on their impact, and whether we choose for this to stay the same, or whether it needs changing.

PART 2:
TRACING THE ROOTS 2

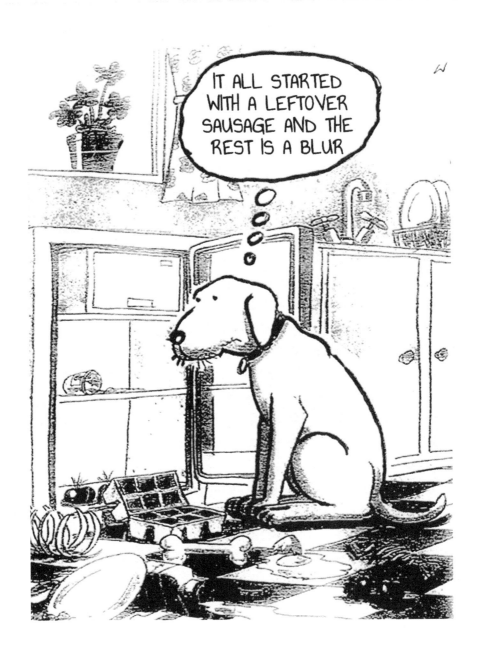

WHAT *ELSE* GETS IN THE WAY?

Moving on from your M.O and how you actually **approach** losing weight, is the myriad of underlying **causes**: our team of triggers and tripwires, if you like.

Have a look through the assortment of areas below for overeating and putting on weight, not being able to lose weight and not holding the weight you are happy with for as long as you would hope.

We will go into each one more fully over the next couple of chapters but this outline will give you an overall idea of the bigger picture.

Where to begin....
The reasons I've listed over the next pages rarely operate on their own but in tandem with some of the others. Part and parcel of knowing where to begin will be by noticing which ones seem to jump out, whether it's a food situation itself or whether overeating is an emotional **end** result. Returning to the image of the swinging metal spheres, cognitive behavioural therapy as it's known, pivots on getting to grips with the circular effect from events or situations in your lives, how they affect what you think and how you feel and how in turn you behave, as in eating behaviour for example... as a result. Except much as with the dog in the picture, it can all happen in the blink of an eye. It's one thing to have enjoyed over indulging, but when our eating behaviour is continually at odds with what we'd planned, we're certainly not at the driving wheel, and as I repeat elsewhere, becoming unaccountable for our behaviour and actions is a real deal breaker in terms of self esteem.

Bearing in mind then that while the common denominator is the need to cut calories and burn off more than you eat, this overstatement of the obvious and getting the balance right is deceptively challenging.

Apart from getting the nutrition you need when trying to "eat less", or when your day is one long rush and the stress is high, apart from manoeuvring your way from one food centred event to another, there's the emotionally addictive element that really adds complexity to the simple matter of nutritionally complete, calorifically restrictive "five a day" ...

Finding the Lead Trigger...

So below are some of the main triggers, in no particular order, that lead to weight gain. You will probably have quite a few amongst these, but finding the one that gets the ball rolling most often is what you want to look for. That one is what I call the **Lead Trigger**, and when things get particularly bad and we're eating for king and country, all the rest come out from under the floorboards to join the party. At that point, it may *feel* as though you're onto a terrible roll of overeating but if you find the main culprit, the rest will calm down or moderate to some extent. Yes, it really is a little like one of those sci-fi programmes where if you hit the android mothership, the rest go down! Incidentally, the lead trigger can be something seemingly benign, but once you're on the look out, noticing your eating behaviours will shine a light on the instigating event! This is where detective work comes in as you follow the "crumb trail" to discover a trigger. It's a kind of treasure hunt in reverse!

Bear in mind it is rare for any of these to be at play on their own. There's usually a mix of two or more which makes for a far more powerful punch and "just simply stopping" a far more tricky manoeuvre. Otherwise we'd have all done it.

UNDERLYING CAUSES:

Food Wisdom – **Lack of Information or Understanding:**
Eating the wrong stuff so massive calorific overload. Maybe it's what you've always done, or maybe you grew into it, either way, if not in tandem with the need for emotional comfort or addictive eating, it could be the easiest one to remedy. In principle anyway!

Physical – **Lack of enough activity:**
Reduced mobility or sat down for hours at work means very little energy burnt off.

For some, recognition is all it takes to rectify, but for many others, easier said than done. Non Exercise Activity Thermogenesis (N.E.A.T) is anything we do other than sleeping which burns off energy. So whether you always mean to do more, or you just hate vigorous movement of the let's get really healthy variety, anything up from zero will be a start.

Physical – **Hormonal or Health issues:**
Health issues or pain management can play havoc not merely with reduced mobility, as above, but with reduced energy for self care if you're cooking for one, and not surprisingly a heightened desire for comfort or reward through food. If your weight has ballooned through steroid induced hunger, your GP will need to monitor this and provide specific support. This may require a huge amount of self compassion, and some very creative problem solving. But it can be done.

Hormonal issues similarly may need at the least to be factored in, or medically monitored and addressed if more disruptive. The good news is that thyroid conditions are now manageable under medication, and other hormonal side effects may simply need an enhanced awareness of the mood swings that precipitate eating behaviours. You may not be able to manage your eating all of the time, but you can work around it a lot of the time or even just part of the month. Again, anything up from zero...

Lifestyle and constraint on time:
Long hours, too much to do, too little time to give thought or effort to good meal planning means food is grabbed, eaten on the run, picking in between, and the rest.

Depending on whether you choose... to overload your life ... or are rather more subject to the demands of work and family combined etc, may dictate the need to get very creative with your planning, or taking a long hard look at what you could delegate or get rid of entirely. Even the smallest thing (something easy) can bring you *back* from a tipping point and the brink of going crazy with the eating.

Lifestyle and communal eating:
Social, work, family, flat sharing, celebrations, event marking, sharing, bonding... an overload of food centred occasions... Bringing this into line usually requires a balance between recognition of what's happening and more conscious choice making. The Rolling Event Calendar may help you through the minefield!

Emotional Eating:

Eating as a reaction to emotions or stress, or to fill a gap of some kind including boredom. Since with the advent of quick fix meals and take-aways, this has slip-slided into our lives as such a panacea for all ills, we often are unaware of just how much we are using food in this way. Discovering which emotions elicit the strongest eating urges often only come to light as we try to reduce the unhealthy eating or drinking. Depending on issues ranging from our historic family eating patterns to things going on here and now in our lives, this is often the slippery customer! But you're worth it!

Automatic eating - 1: Bad habits

Unconscious eating – eating as a habit: any or all of the above combined and now happening on its own. Whether highly complex or mundane in the extreme, none of us are exempt from this, but Trigger Tracking and finding ways to override the Automatic Impulse, (aka habit,) promotes tremendous psychological muscle power and self possession. A bit like cracking the Enigma Code, it can actually be immensely rewarding with long lasting results!

Automatic eating - 2: The Food Addict

Highly compulsive and unconscious eating and often resilient to change – **highly addictive eating**: even assuming you recognise all of the above, you simply can't stop eating. It's like it's hardwired somehow in your brain. Unless you are in denial you could well be feeling completely helpless and out of control.

Whilst recognising where and how and why your eating behaviour is happening, greater support and other approaches rather than cognitive or behavioural ones alone may be needed. Although recognition and insight will be essential, this level of addiction may have nothing to do with how much willpower you do or don't possess.

It operates from a totally different area of the brain, and can respond well to the kind of treatment that is used for trauma recovery, such as Eye

Movement Desensitisation Remedy, (EMDR)[10] and Somatic Experiencing[11] or some types of work involving NLP (Neuro Linguistic Programming)[12] and guided visualisation. We are familiar with the concepts of fight or flight, but the "freeze" mode of survival - now linked with more intensely addictive behaviours as well as trauma - is often beneath a behaviour pattern here that just keeps replaying.

This said, an intense emotional trigger can easily masquerade in the same way, so if you are clinically to morbidly obese, don't jump to conclusions before you've looked at the in depth chapter on Emotional Eating. I have clients who have lost 15 stone and kept the weight off, so there is always hope!!

Most of the detective work you'll be doing is in finding out what happens in the *gap* between what we meant to do when we got up in the morning and what we actually did by the time we went to bed. We're effectively Minding the Gap.

Minding the Gap is the bit that joins the dots between needing something to do, needing something to be entertained by, something to stimulate the senses, and needing something which gives us focus; something equally which fills the bit that the need for comfort or relief leaves open, and something with which to mark time, to break up the day, and provides meaning and tradition to our lives. We need to join those dots.

Whether you're overeating to your cost for pleasurably social reasons,

---

[10] EMDR: A therapy developed by Francine Shapiro that works to alleviate symptoms of trauma.

[11] Somatic Experiencing is a form of therapy aimed at relieving and resolving the symptoms of post-traumatic stress disorder (PTSD) and other mental and physical trauma-related health problems by focusing on the client's perceived body sensations (or somatic experiences).

[12] Neuro-linguistic programming (NLP) created by Richard Bandler and John Grinder in the 1970s. Its creators claim a connection between the neurological processes ("neuro"), language ("linguistic") and behavioral patterns learned through experience ("programming") and that these can be changed to achieve specific goals in life.

or whether it's poly-filling gaps in your emotional world and doing rather too good a job at that, coming away from anything which has had benefits, hidden or otherwise, is not the easiest thing to do but remember that even with the smallest steps, **Change happens Fast!!** We can often feel entirely different about ourselves or our situation within hours of taking even a part of it in hand!! Even if your actual eating behaviour or capacity for self sabotage is causing you as much angst as your weight, you have choice: You can choose to take one small step today, knowing you are doing the best you can at any given moment.

I am though, going to take a closer look at **Habit** first, because it really is the superglue that keeps things stuck, even when the original reason has long since lost relevance and been forgotten.

...Anything up from zero is a good enough place to start...!

REASONS FOR OVEREATING...

HABIT: The Automatic Impulse and Unconscious Behaviour...

HABIT: The Automatic Impulse and Unconscious Behaviour...

One of the overriding reasons for drifting off track, and this frequently applies to long term weight holding as much as the initial weight loss itself, is life getting in the way and that wonderful old nugget, habit. I take most of the book exploring where and how it most holds, and of course, how to cut the bind, but key to this intent, however oft we fail or flounder, is recognition.

If a new habit is the untrod path with hidden pitfalls and little light, it takes little to imagine the pull back to the familiar: the old habit is like a well worn motorway that makes the same old route an over easy option, and the hardest part often enough is that everything that contributes to our environment, what we do, the impact on our feelings and energy levels, all combine to keep it securely in place.

The purpose of the following three chapters is to look at how, when, where and why they are kept in place within the fabric of our lifestyles, and what triggers them emotionally or physically. Instrumental in keeping us stuck however, is our underestimating their tenacity, and not factoring it in. It is **because** of the resilience of habit to change, that we need to take so much time, not only knowing where they most hold in relation to our eating behaviours and patterns, but *recognising* where they fall between habit on the one hand, and *addiction* on the other.

Should you... by the way... recoil at the use of the "A" word, which surely must only refer to substance or alcohol addiction, take a look at the definition below:

"A degree of involvement in a behaviour that can function both to produce pleasure and to provide relief from discomfort, to the point where the costs appear to outweigh the benefits."

(McMurran 1994[13])

---

[13] The Psychology of Addiction by Mary McMurran – Taylor and Francis 1994

Ring any bells?

Let's look too at a Guideline for Addictive Behaviour[14] and see whether that also sounds familiar:

- Denying your behaviour is cause for concern

- Telling yourself repeatedly that:

- I won't eat/drink like this after today

- This is the last time

- I'll start again tomorrow

- I am doing this because…. (Insight as the excuse..!)

- Defensiveness and irritation with others about food / weight issues

- Plans and good intentions not working

So….Habit or Addiction? The silent spectrum…

Good habits, bad habits, leading to seriously entrenched habits and levels of addiction, the question is when *does* plain old habit become a hard and fast addiction?

Habit	Serious habit	Addiction

There's an ocean covering the spectrum holding habit at the one end and addiction at the other. The point at which we keep reverting back to default, falling, if not catapulting ourselves down that same hole in the road, will indeed be the pointer. Some of the descriptions below might resonate:

THE AUTOMATIC PILOT…
THE AUTOMATIC IMPULSE…
THE UNCONSCIOUS IMPULSE…

[14] Guidelines for Addictive Behaviour - groupwork module - www.lighterlife.co.uk

UNCONSCIOUS BEHAVIOUR...
WILD MONKEY / NOT NORMAL SELF... at the driving wheel...

I've gone a tad overboard and given several names to the above because while everybody recognizes the existence of habits, few people initially recognize its power. I see this regularly when someone who has conquered mountains in terms of portion control and generally reactive eating... is devastated to discover that once they have settled at a happy enough weight, the old patterns still creep back in. And predictably, if you do what you did before, you'll get what you had before. It's why I have usually found a person who is on their third or fourth run, really starts to get it. The frustration is being advised often with vehemence that a person is doing the wrong diet.

Of course the diet *may* be at fault. A "diet", if you can call it that, high in sugar and processed carbohydrates (i.e. cake, biscuits, bread etc) *is* addictive. Far more often though, it is the *impulse* which is overwhelming. Being *ahead of the habit,* or overriding it with a new, more appealing distraction, is where the work lies, *as well* as changing what's being eaten.

The return of a few old ways may not be such a concern but it's when you begin to have that old feeling of slowly losing control that it gets upsetting, then scary. Losing power and personal accountability makes anyone feel helpless and vulnerable. But it's the level of surprise and shock that people have – like swimming in a tide that turns out to have a far stronger undertow than one ever imagined, that gives the game away. It's the strength of what I call the **Automatic Impulse** that is unexpected for the most part. And as I mentioned it takes people quite a few attempts to realise what they're up against. So yet again, *recognition* is key.

The word "habit" often has bad press because of our extraordinary skill in accumulating bad ones, but we have a lot of good habits too: stuff we do again and again and again... (apparently it takes only six repetitions to create a habit but the undoing of one with a lot of benefits, such as overeating, can be much more laboured!!) and is often coupled, or "anchored in", with an action, a place, a person... Think cinema and popcorn, TV and dinner, drinks and canapés or cigarettes. It's a minefield.

More positively, look at the repeat practice for anything you want to excel in, such as our Olympian participants. They would have "built up" as they call it, for months prior to the event and probably years before. It's basic physiology coupled in their case with sufficient talent which enables them increasingly to rely on a base level of expertise.

Further, when you practice anything, enough, it becomes instinctive, hard wired into the reflexes of our musculature. The untrod road becomes the new motorway. When things go wrong – quite often it is because our mind has got in the way.

Hence the advent in past years of Sports Psychology. Never was that adage "Let go of your mind and come to your senses," so apt. When we have repeated an action, or a way of thinking, enough, it becomes part of a neural pathway... and rather like a motorway with its regular usage, our quickest route to somewhere. We fall on the familiar, and the easiest road to somewhere, again and again, and again. It's what we're designed to do, it's automatic, and it's the path of least resistance. The problem of course, with less desirable habits being that we have indeed let go of our minds, but our senses are ruling the roost. The tail is wagging the dog!

Just to demonstrate this at its most basic, at a level of physiological reflex, cast your mind to the last time you moved home or office. Can you recall reaching to switch on a light that is not in that place but WAS where you previously lived or worked? It can carry on for weeks before you stop reaching up, automatically, for the old place. Unlike a second helping of food or a bar of chocolate, there is no emotional reward in reaching for the old place. There is no family history or underlying agenda. No gratification of the senses. It's just a reflex which has settled in and will take time for the new habit to replace. So it shouldn't take too much of a leap to appreciate the pull of something which *does* contain an alluring reward: does have an immediate, here and now gratification or an enjoyable mood altering effect.

You can imagine what a potent package that bar of chocolate is, or whatever we're reaching for. The prevailing problem with food, is that whilst we can survive with**out** alcohol or cigarettes, (though you may not *feel* like that...) we *cannot* survive without food. We are required as it were to retain enough of the "habit" to nourish ourselves appropriately, without going the whole lock, stock and barrel.

We need the hair of the dog... but not the whole coat...

The **positive function** of a habit then, is indeed part of our survival kit. If we had to remember everything, from new, each time anew, we'd never get past first base on anything. Part of our ability to manage information so that we then have space for other, new stuff, is based on our ability to store information and retrieve it at will, as the need arises. In this respect, habit is hard to get a grip on because it works behind the scenes, but it is *meant* to work behind the scenes.

This applies physically as well as mentally. If you think how we learn to walk, and have to "re-learn" if we have a stroke or an accident which prevents the brain sending its message to parts of our body. Equally, accumulating knowledge as we increase in familiarity means that we progress. If you recall maybe learning to drive... or anything which was initially laboured but is now easy... you start off as the white knuckled new kid on the block... all brain cells focussed on the task yet within months will accomplish the same route in a state of relative absent mindedness...

The process of learning from scratch to being fully competent and doing something without thinking underpins what is called the "Four Stages of Learning"[15] and our capacity to form habits. The same habits which unknowingly gain their grip and graft as unerringly to parts of our nervous reflex system, as our emotional "need" to have whatever it supposedly provides.

The fact is no one is immune from habit, since to be alive and well relies at its most basic upon an autonomous system which instinctively performs without our thinking about it. Automatic pilot, as with reaching for the switch, is as normal as breathing.

So too, is unconscious behaviour, the effect of which is no less binding

---

[15] The Four Stages of Learning - Abraham Maslow 1940. Sometimes known as the Four Stages of Competency, goes from what we didn't know we didn't know – to what we know so well we now do without thinking: Unconscious Incompetence; Conscious Incompetence; Conscious Competence; Unconscious Competence.

than the tug of an undercurrent which can pull the strongest swimmer off their feet to their peril.

The key though, is to factor it in, and not underestimate its pull and power.

I am as pedantic beyond belief in my labouring the minutia of our habit making process as I have been with the varying stages of motivation, because it gets overlooked, again and again. Expecting a newly formed eating regime to simply stay there once we've achieved the weight loss we want, is like expecting your most mischievous mongrel pet to stay put when there is no longer a reward. Our beloved pet needs training as well as the reassurance that a different reward is on its way. Or put another way, we understand that if we train for a sport, it takes time, and moreover, continued practise. We don't expect to produce a rabbit out of the hat. That ten foot hurdle needs time and effort and a massive amount of motivation to bother in the first place.

The easy bit about a ten foot hurdle on the playing ground however, is that at least it's out there. By contrast the *impulse* to overeat comes seemingly unbidden from within. It is always said that you can't solve a problem from the mindset that created it, but in one sense, trying to leave behind old habits with such a great benefits package other than getting fat, is exactly that. It means we need a very stealthy approach to enable our way through the mire. If you think of David Attenborough tiptoeing his way through the undergrowth, it's a lot like that.

Spotting the habit *making* to enable habit *breaking!*
In their (very readable) book on Mindfulness[16], Professor Mark Williams and Dr Danny Penman say that habit breaking is straightforward. It is, but it's breaking ones with a built in comfort factor and a resistance to letting go, that can be problematic. It's also assuming we are "mindful" of where and when those habits keep reoccurring.

Heightening your awareness as to where and when they keep

---

[16] Mindfulness: A practical guide to finding peace in a frantic world by Prof Mark Williams & Dr Danny Penman. PIATKUS – May 2011

happening, and understanding better what lies beneath, will help to soften their hold.

Generally, it's a three pronged approach:

Recognition, motivation and strategy...
The first absolutely has to be a ***recognition*** of where and how your eating habits have most hold, together with a ***recognition*** of the durability and tenaciousness of those habits. It's deeply upsetting, infuriating and frustrating when the old roots come back again and again to make our lives hell. But rather like the world's most resilient knotweed, or your favourite mole digging up a lawn without a soupçon of care for your feelings, that's what they do. Expecting this not to happen is like wishing for Santa Claus. Knowing it will happen unless you do something different means you've started training.

The second is ***motivation***, with long term motivation being the nut that can be so hard to crack.

The third, which might be a work in progress for the more ingrained habits, is about ***strategy,*** and finding ways to work with them. Some will be easier to let go of, and I will always go there first, though that will vary from person to person. Others need a more cunning approach to be sidestepped or appeased... This is where strategy comes in.

Caroline Myss suggests that the struggle with addiction "may well be one of the foremost defining health challenges of our age"[17]. The almost exponential increase in obesity and the recent inclusion of binge eating disorder in medical manuals[18] bears testimony to this. It makes sense that

---

[17] Addiction: Explored as an Archetypal Journey Toward Personal Empowerment – Caroline Myss / CMED Institute 27/06/2011 -
www.myss.com/CMED/workshops/addiction

[18] Although not yet included as an addiction, the inclusion of Binge Eating Disorder as a diagnostic category in DSM-V (The American Psychiatric Association – May 2013) "bodes well for the eventual recognition of food addiction as a substance use disorder in future editions of the manual." FAI (Food Addiction Inst. 08/2013)

part of the way through, is to be *ahead* of the habit. Recognition as to how, and when, and where it takes root, and gathers strength, must soon be an essential "need to know" of our wellbeing and survival.

Indeed simply **noticing**, bringing any overeating habit into more vivid awareness, plucks it out of where it has been hiding. It starts to take away the strength of that automatic impulse that acts without thinking. *Noticing*, then, for the many who despair as to what they can do, is *already doing something.*

For now, from the social to the emotional, let's take a look at the hidey hole of some of those eating habits:

Life,
Stuff,
and the
Socially Driven Spectrum

LIFE, STUFF and the SOCIALLY DRIVEN SPECTRUM...

The whole point of the Social spectrum is to provide you with an immediately visible map. This map will hold information as to where you go, what you do, who with, in other words a tangible trail of your day, any day of the week, any week of the year. It's layer numero uno of your *Eating Behaviour Blueprint.*

Whilst rearranging any of your timetables or routines as a strategy to sidestepping pitfalls may be a task in itself, it's a lot simpler than trying to moderate emotions, which are not so easily put in a box.

That's why it's essential that changes you look to put into place early on are *easy*: it's the Montessori[19] principle whereby whatever you tackle is always doable, and always meaningful, however small. This way, you start out knowing you can do it, it gets done, and you have a sense of achievement. By the time it gets to the more challenging stuff, you're already more confident and in a better headspace. Starting from easy puts you onto a win-win from the outset.

A great example if you drive, is changing when you get petrol. This isn't usually a problem as it's quick, so unless you're returning from night shift or have had a horribly late night, you are **less** likely to go for the goodies on the counter on the way to work than you are when you're tired and maybe stressed later in the day. An exception however, of snacking at the morning fill up, was a new mother whose baby kept her up at all hours. Mums take note!

The same goes for the time you go shopping but depending on your circumstances this could get a tad more complicated: even people who don't use food to console are far more likely to indulge when they are cold and tired and hungry. However it can be slightly more of an issue to do this earlier on if you work: where *is* all that food going to go during the day?? Can you get someone else who isn't as tempted to buy treats early evening to do the shopping instead, assuming you trust whoever it is to get the right stuff... etc etc...? You can see already that although this can

---

[19] Maria Montessori 1870 – 1952: An Italian physician best known for the philosophy on education which bears her name.

be easy enough to implement, and you could of course shop online, there's more to it.

As you add the details of your lifestyle and environment into your personal map you're basically keeping an eye out for what **can** be changed, to best effect. Changing and maintaining new eating behaviours can already be difficult enough without adding to the challenge: so aim at all times to look for minimal effort, maximum impact! Your approach will benefit however from being methodical, and generating new routines to replace the dangerous ones. Do not think you can operate "off the cuff" or on a "see how it goes" basis, as that operating behind the scenes monkey, which lest you forget is you later in the day… will simply get the upper hand. Whatever you do, planning is pivotal. Our emotions are less predictable, but taking charge of circumstances to the extent you are able will have a massively beneficial effect **on** the emotions. If you're a late nighter, and perpetually slightly tired or worse for wear the following day from alcohol, it's an uphill battle not to dip into something comforting come later in the day. Getting to bed an hour or so earlier is most likely your best chance of maintaining focus and resolve with your eating habits.

So managing a lot of this with military precision, as it's the one area you **can** apply military position, will really work in your favour.

Apart from being tidy, it means you're going to feel a whole lot more certain of yourself when the going gets tough. But hopefully you get the idea….

….planning is pivotal to the plot…..

EATING BEHAVIOURS: THE NEED FOR STRUCTURE AND MEANING

Time and event related eating.

Lifestyle and all its extenuating circumstances provide the framework in which our need for comfort exists. It also largely dictates the extent to which we have these needs and what they might be. For instance if stress levels are high, our time limited, and we are constantly overtired, we might desire a healthier more active lifestyle but end up all too often opting for peace and quiet and a take-away in front of the TV. Conversely if we have far more time on our hands, a looser structure to our daily lives, we often choose to eat to pass the time. So already, the impact of the structures we create or are subject to in our lives is easy to see.

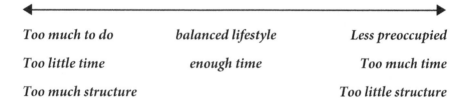

Too much to do	*balanced lifestyle*	*Less preoccupied*
Too little time	*enough time*	*Too much time*
Too much structure		*Too little structure*

It's often cited you eat to live, you don't live to eat. At the very least, the sustenance it provides on a daily level adds another basic structure to our lives. On top of which, the notion of elevenses or tea time gives not merely an energy boost to take us past a part of the day, when having been up since dawn our sugar levels start to dip, but moreover a mini milestone in time. It breaks the day whether we are working, at home or on holiday, into manageable and more enjoyable portions. Meal breaks, beverage breaks, snacks, any moment, in fact, we stop to eat or drink anything, however small, is like syntax to the sentence, interspersing and shifting the tempo of our day, whether to pass the time or alleviate the tedium, often as not with a great big full stop at the end.

Capping it all, in a way that is pervasive to our species, eating provides communion: a way of sharing, whether intimately, as a family, as a central point for bonding and interacting professionally, or indeed as part of a more traditional or sacred rite of passage such as the wedding or bar mitzvah feast. To paraphrase the Marks and Spencer's adverts – this... is not just a way of keeping ourselves alive, this... is memory making in action, this... has meaning, chicken soup for the soul and so on.

The beauty of this, as well as the worry, is that in eating terms, we have 3 or more times a day, 365 days of the year, which provide such opportunity.

Because so much eating is emotionally driven and therefore quite elusive, I find it less daunting to begin with the more practical approach, hence starting out with the Social Spectrum, and hence too my propensity for list making.

More importantly, by separating the lists into What, When, Why, Where and Who, it brings to light the elements of a situation which are problematic, or not. Further, by creating your own lists so that they become effectively, page at a glance, it's in yer face, to use an undignified expression, giving you less room to wriggle but ultimately more information for better choice making.

Have a look at the lists on the following pages and complete your own, however you prefer, adding your own dates and events. You will see they fall into various categories differentiating types of event, their times and their meanings. The point in looking at the meaning of an event is that when you come to adding the whole lot up – you'll start to notice those which have high value from those which have become more of a habit and hold less value. When you begin to "budget" what you imbibe, and see your eating as ranging from "emotionally and / or socially valuable" to "wasted calories" – which is the equivalent of dropping coins through a hole in the pocket – this will help you decide which "events" you can more easily let go of in the future, or at least shift from being food related in some way, to some other focus.

The **what** is either the meal or the event which may vary from being food and drink centred, to less directly related, but food and drink is still in there somewhere.

The **when** obviously relates to its timing.

The **why** relates to the level of meaning it has for us and what that is.

THE WHAT...	THE WHEN...	THE WHY...
Meals	*Times*	*Meaning*
	How long between meal times?	
	How late is the last meal?	
Breakfast		
Elevenses / Coffee break		
Lunch	Time of day	Personal
Tea break		Professional
Snacking / picking / grazing…		
	Time of night	
Light Dinner	Time of the week:	
Heavy Dinner	weekday / weekend	
	Time of month / year	

Food or drink centred events

		Habitual
Work related		Seasonal
		Ritual
Personal –	Actual dates	Intimate
Birthdays		Celebrating
Anniversaries		Commemorating
Weddings		
Christenings		
Funerals		Rite of Passage
National holidays		
Religious holidays		
Bank holidays		Traditional
Personal holidays		

You can start from the most basic – noting first your regular meal times, whether they're small or large as a rule, and include all the regular snacking or picking times in between.

For example, if you are the person doing the cooking, and you are eating all the leftovers, one of your examples might go:

THE WHAT...	THE WHEN...	THE WHY...
Picking at leftovers cooking for family at lunch / dinner	7pm...9pm etc	habitual

Especially if you are someone who is fine until you get home from work, or fine until you start - at which point you seem to continue, note down whether you go a long time between meals so that you really *are* over hungry.

Note down also how *late* your last meal is, particularly if it is a large or heavy meal. You may not be able to do much about the timing if you tend to get in late, but you can *what* you eat and make sure it is lighter.

Notice and write down how often you buy the "bogof"s (buy one get one free). If dieting costs you extra, buying freebies is hardly an economy if you eat them all: it's yet another risk of temptation coming wrapped as a saving.

Write down how many times a day you have to cook, and if for example you have a habit of eating the leftovers. Your meals are *habitual* but your eating the leftovers is a *habit.*

By differentiating between whether something is just a habit, which has no meaning, or a ritual, which may or may not be necessary but does hold some meaning, you'll begin to get a sense of how much could, in theory anyway, be dropped!

Using and expanding on these examples, complete your own list over page, making clear what the meaning holds for you personally.

YOUR EATING BEHAVIOUR BLUEPRINT
THE SOCIALLY DRIVEN SPECTRUM

THE WHAT...	*THE WHEN...*	*THE WHY...*
Meals	**Times**	**Meaning**
Snacking / picking / grazing...		
Food / drink related events		
-		
-		
-		
-		
-		
-		
-		
-		
-		
-		
-		
-		
-		
-		
-		
-		

Ask yourself:

What do you find most difficult?

When do you typically find it most difficult?

What exactly happens? What are each of the steps leading to a typical overeating pattern?

-

-

-

-

-

Is the overeating: The food itself i.e. take-aways, junk food, high calorie etc...?

- Lack of portion control?
- Picking between meal times?
- Using up b.o.g.o.fs (buy one get one free)

How much of the eating, or food, do you suspect might be unnecessary?

-

-

-

How much of it could be dropped, left out, stopped?

-

-

-

Which do you believe might be the easiest to stop?

-

-

-

Which would be the hardest?

-

-

-

Can you reschedule things for when you're not tired or hungry? Not so vulnerable to temptation? For example shopping, filling up with petrol etc.

Could you shop online and avoid the supermarkets when you're tired?

*Can you make sure you don't go for such a long stretch without eating in the afternoon and so do **not** get over hungry? I.e. have something small between 1pm and 5pm, and take the wolf from the door before you go into overdrive.*

How might you do that?

***What** could you have?*

When?

-

-

-

-

-

-

I would recommend that even when you have filled in as much as you can, make a larger chart and put it somewhere visible, so anytime you remember something you overlooked, you can add it in. This can be on your iPhone or on the wall. The point is it gets seen and hence used, regularly. Again, we are appealing as much to the Wild Monkey on Automatic Pilot as the rational part of your brain which makes normal decisions! While it differs from your "most wanted" list earlier on, it acts none the less as a reminder to factor in on a daily basis. Moreover, the effort we make to do this in itself cannot but filter, however slowly or silently, into the less conscious side of ourselves which all too often acts against our better judgement. Anyone who watched Derren Brown in the episode[20] where he predicted what two advertising guys would sketch on a drawing board, will have seen just how much we take in every single bit of our environment without our knowing. This is the bit we are aiming at. This is the bit that gets underestimated, over and again, and finds 90% of dieters wondering despairingly how they could lose the eating - even just a tiny bit less - weight management plot, quite so easily.

Layers of meaning…
The idea of creating these lists is to be able to choose when and where eating is superfluous to requirement and could be dropped!! Often this is too difficult in the first instance either because it's too much of a habit, or too tempting, or the occasion or situation makes it awkward. But there *will* be areas which, once flagged up, you will find are easily dropped.

One of the most useful ways of these areas coming to light is by differentiating between the mindless and the meaningful.

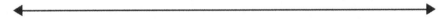

Mindless eating/drinking   *Meaningful eating/drinking*

Cast your mind to situations where you typically wished you didn't drink or pick so much, as well as those where the eating was socially and emotionally valuable:

-

-

-

-

-

-

---

[20] Derren Brown: Subliminal Advertising episode – Sept 2006

Be careful not to rush to a predictable judgement: one person mindlessly munching day and night in front of the TV might be very different to someone else whose TV dinner offers serious downtime and is restorative. In this respect, go through your lists and assign them high or low emotional value where it's relevant. Ask yourself always: is my eating emotionally or socially valuable? Even on your own, it can hold emotional value: some communities regard all food intake as sacred. So equally, you might ask yourself: is whatever I am eating, and how I choose to eat it, sacred, or are they wasted, throwaway calories.

All of this starts to put a very illuminating dot on the "i"…

◄───►

Wasted calories	Socially and / or Emotionally valuable
Throwaway calories	Sacred calories
Meaningless eating	Meaningful eating
Mindless	Mindful
Unconscious eating	Conscious eating

For example, if you regularly go out with the girls or the lads on a Friday or Saturday night, on a mundane level it's just a night out. But if you start to unpick the layers, a deeper meaning unfolds: in the first place it has merit because it marks the end of a working week, and you want to *relax* and be entertained, as much as you feel the right to *reward* yourself.

Over and above that however, it might also represent a *ritual* event that marks the bonds of friendship, and may even *identify* you with a particular group or clan.

Whilst this might be more in evidence with younger people who may feel more pressured to align with their peers, it is none the less present at any age: whether it's the pub after football or rugby matches, party night with the girls, a stag do with the guys, or yet another person's birthday at work with yet another string of cakes to mark the moment, *not joining in* might have to be done with great subtlety to avoid making a statement you don't intend. And that's assuming you are even able to resist temptation. You can see how the plot starts to thicken. But I'll be stirring the pot with emotional factors and what we think and believe might be going on... a little later.

Similarly, Sunday lunch is often a ritual for a family gathering that keeps time apart especially for that purpose. For many people it's the one time in the week they can come together in this way so is almost sacrosanct and holds high importance. But you've got the picture by now so start hand picking those examples.

Not that important	*v*	*emotionally / socially valuable*
-		
-		
-		
-		
-		
-		

The next bit we are going to add into the melting pot is **Where:**

For some people, being out of sight is when they are most likely to eat in secret. For others, it might be eating in the car or on public transport. It's fascinating how many of us fail to factor in the calories eaten on the run, as if they don't count. If only!! Often as well, the "where" is exacerbated by the "when", such as having to run the gauntlet through a main station strewn with eateries when late, tired or over hungry!

Or as an example of the monumentally mundane yet unbelievably hard to stop, is the never ending run of treats or birthday bits left compellingly in view in the open office: the urge to indulge just about held in check till a predictable energy dip later in the day... here the "where" as in "full view", combined with the "when" of "all day", meets its nemesis come tea time.

As the timing combination is most often of equal relevance – I've also added a "**When**" column.

WHERE:	WHEN:
Examples…	Examples…
Outside – restaurants, cafes, shopping malls, fetes	Mealtimes Between mealtimes Early / late in day…
In the home: In the kitchen	Some of the day? At vulnerable times in the day?
At work: In the canteen or kitchen At your desk On a visible place too within reach in an open plan office	Just tea breaks Most of the day
Your route outward bound / home etc: In the car - short routine journeys In the car – long journeys	Once a week, Twice a week, Daily etc
On the train	How often Morning, evening etc
In a hospital	Visiting times etc

-

-

-

-

-

-

Ask yourself:

*Where **are** you whenever you succumb to temptation?*

*As both sight and smell lowers the resistance, where have you **been**?*

*As anticipation equally counts – where are you **going**?*

Are you near food a lot of the time?

Does your route somewhere take you past a lot of food outlets, stalls, cafes etc?

-

Do you have to run the gauntlet past all the food temptations at a mainline station?

-

*With the two preceding questions, how **long** does it generally take?*

Does it coincide with being genuinely (over?) hungry?

If so, can you have something small and less lethal to tide you through, beforehand?

If with the same two questions, you are not in fact hungry, and especially if the route is not a long one, could you bolster yourself head down, eyes on the ground, and get through unscathed?

If not, could you change your route?

When is your worst time of day?

If you are in an open plan office with snack food forever in sight, could you:

- Ask that it's only there during the break times.
- Ask that it's moved to the kitchen or lounge if either exists… (Remember it's a work environment, not a café for heaven's sake!)
- Suggest for Health and Safety that a cover is put over the offending items. It's less to do with hygiene mind, and more to do with not being visibly assailed with merciless continuity till the dip in the day when you give in. Though for real effectiveness the

dome like cover does need to be non transparent. I jest not. Millions spent on advertising attests to the power of visual stimulus. Out of sight seriously bolsters the resistance. *Act* on it.

If you spend a lot of the time in the kitchen, and that contributes to unnecessary snacking, can you spend less time in there?

If you are finishing off all the remains of whatever you serve, on a regular basis, can you: buy and cook less, (there's a thought!)?

Immediately dispose with leftovers or drizzle with washing up liquid? Fast.

If for example, the kitchen is a large room so you use it as an office or recreationally, can you move to another room?

Can you rearrange the trigger foods in your kitchen so they are higher up, or at the back of shelves, more out of sight and less immediately reachable?

Lastly, we'll add **Who** into the equation.

Who we are with also makes a difference.

Many people with a visible weight issue say that in public, and especially in company, they are in fact more likely to control their eating as they fear what others might be thinking and being judged. Conversely, others find the smorgasbord of visible offerings too hard to resist, or are more tempted to *reward* themselves when sharing a meal with others.

If you're on a diet at your best friend's wedding which to boot you committed to months before, she just might take umbrage if you open your cuppa NoCal soup at the main banquet, especially if it's a sit down affair. On the other hand, if you're with a slightly controlling friend who always insists you have pie and paella even when you're not actually hungry, you can see how this is a world apart. The situations we are in, where, when and with whom, all add up to affecting that inner calculus which operates without a moment's thought, and affects our eating behaviour. At the least, upping the awareness starts to put us *back in charge!!* Less of the *Wild Monkey!*

Ask yourself:

Who tends to have a bad influence on you?

Is this because you don't assert yourself?

Is it because they sabotage you?

Is it because you want to have fun / belong and be part of whatever's going on?

Do you find yourself too easily distracted with certain people?

What other reasons?

-

-

-

-

-

-

If you're not sure, notice what happens when next in their company.

-

Can you rearrange to see people whose company is too conducive to overeating, at a different time?

Combining *the situations with the when and the who and the where...*

List your best or trickiest examples:

-

-

-

-

-

-

List examples that come up repeatedly:

Remember What, When, Why, Where, Who?

-

-

-

-

-

Intensifying your awareness with regard to when and where you overeat, who with and the type of situation, will enable you increasingly to make choices ahead of the event. Whether that "event" is mindless picking with a glass in your hand before dinner, or whether it's more public, doesn't matter: what matters is that you notice more and more and that you begin by making the changes you can rely upon. Which is why keeping to small, doable shifts in your eating patterns is all that matters at the start. Looking at your lists, if something has a high meaning in terms of the why, it might be less easy to change and you may not wish to change it. Go for something of low value and ideally one that isn't accompanied by a high stress factor, though we'll be looking at that later.

From this first layer of your Eating Behaviour Blueprint, what changes could you make very quickly?

-

-

-

-

-

Remember:
What do you ***want?***
What are you ***willing to do?***
What are you ***able to do?***

Make your lists as full and comprehensive and as relevant as you can, add to them, whenever, and we'll use them as reference throughout the Emotional and Physical overeating spectrums as well.

We'll be doing this and asking some of the same questions after each chapter.

The idea is that as we combine the Social, the Emotional and the Physically driven spectrums, a much clearer picture of your eating behaviour patterns and how and why things have historically gone off track will manifest almost magically before your eyes. Hopefully there'll be a few light bulb moments over and above the glaringly obvious. Though again, the obvious is never obvious enough, otherwise you'd have had it sorted long ago.

The SOCIAL SPECTRUM and the impact of CULTURE

The banner of "Social" encompasses lifestyle, situations, circumstance etc, and within this not just your immediate environment, i.e. where you live and with whom... but the wider backdrop of your culture and heritage.

Wherever you come from, your values and beliefs are part and parcel of your history, but as I mentioned in "Do You *Need* to Lose Weight," getting a handle on how this influences your ideas about food and size and weight will put you one step ahead.

CULTURAL LEGACY:

Time was... when having weight indicated affluence, and hence better health to boot. Many people still associate health and even survival, with extra pounds, or weight loss by contrast with illness and death. It can be a conundrum if you prefer a western slimness but come from a community where weight is akin to good health and background. If you are caught in this... a good look at health issues rather than image and aesthetics... might keep you on a safer track. Can you associate slimness with health and vitality? If your cholesterol is shooting through the ceiling along with your blood pressure and your family have a history of weight related diabetes etc, that'll be a gauge to keep your weight in balance. You're still left with mastering temptation and the eating habits of a lifetime mind, but at least you'll not be kidding yourself that the extra weight is good, or a survival need - and knowing what you want and intend – is the first step.

CULTURAL ISSUES:

My Mum's Italian / Indian / Muslim / Jewish...

Welcome to the world!! Most of us, if we are lucky anyway, had a specific someone whose job it was to feed us. For many of us too, if that was a nourishing experience, emotionally as well as physically, it's incredibly tempting to go back for more. To draw a line however, and neutralize a potential minefield of discrimination, let's just say that there can be mums / women / people... of any race, creed and class who might over feed. Who will see their providing ample fare as a statement of the love they offer, the prestige they hold, or how good they are as a person / mum /

145

wife / matriarch / head of family etc etc... and by virtue of this your dieting... or watching your weight... as a statement of rejection of their love, or that they are not good enough. The archetypically domineering mother who uses "nurturing" as a benefit with strings and conditions attached, can indeed be very difficult if it's combined with liking food a bit too much anyway. If in addition, refusing food or at least a second or third helping is tantamount to rejection or rudeness... and add *that* to finding it difficult to resist as well... it gets even more complicated and packs a potent punch. Probably safe to say that if your family and extended family is... very extended, the cooking scenario can be a real issue... Sustained willpower doesn't usually cut it when you're the main person cooking, so getting canny and working around temptation will be particularly relevant. Probably the best way to elicit family support will be to pull the "health card", but see later in "Working the System" for more inspiration!

FAMILY HISTORY AND LEARNT BEHAVIOUR PATTERNS:

Similar to the above in some ways, but here the eating behaviour is unique to the family. Often we look for biological or genetic dispositions, and they do exist[21] [22], but equally prevalent are behaviours and responses and reactions that are passed down the generations without apparent notice. If you are human, and alive, you will have these – it's just that some of the learnt behaviours are beneficial, and some plain ain't. Eating junk foods or overeating are not great in the long run. One of the difficulties is not merely the addiction to sugar or wheat or fries or whatever, but also the fact it can be wrapped up with an identity: "This is what we do or how we share good times or show love in our family. This is how we look. It's our modus operandi." To do something different can feel like, or be taken as, a rejection or a statement of superiority. It's worth remembering that before the availability of fast foods plus the throw back to post war thrift, bags of crisps and such like were rarely bought or left around for casual indulgence.

---

[21] The Genetics of Obesity in Adult Adoptees and their Biological Siblings:
T.I.Sorensen, R.A. Price, A.J. Stunkard and F. Schulsinger - BMJ 14th Jan 1982
[22] The Genetics of Obesity: T.I. Sorensen Sept 1995

FAMILY HISTORY AND GENETIC OBESITY:

Statistically on the increase and, with a propensity for obesity in the offspring of the obese themselves, very concerning. Continuing from the discovery of a "fat gene" in the eighties, the genetics / environment interaction shows a marked increase within what is ironically termed a "favourable" environment, given a pre existing family history. Since that very (obesogenic) environment is currently affecting thousands of us with no such background, it's not exactly good news. Studies are ever ongoing and it makes fascinating reading[23] but for the meantime, there seems no definitive answer other than being informed, and choosing to take action sooner rather than later if you or your family come under this banner. That choice may be a lifestyle which more actively promotes physical and emotional health; nutritional balance, which may include the omission, for the greater part, of crave inducing foods (see Food Wisdom and curbing the urge chapter) and keeping one step ahead of eating behaviours. But at least that choice is there. The "fat gene" thus describes a *tendency* to gain weight – but need not be a foregone conclusion.

What might be of importance here, if your body *naturally* rests above what is deemed a healthy weight, is not to succumb to the "what's the point" or "it's not fair" school of despondency and end up overeating to comfort yourself. Some people simply have what is called a higher set point[24], but providing you keep an eye on your health, (and your girth,) providing you are not showing signs of weight related diabetes or suchlike, then work to stay where you *are*. Don't let your *mind*set play hell with your weight set!

Another factor which can appear down the generations relates to the effects of the dopamine, or reward centre of the brain. A propensity for addiction has been found to run through families – studies proving an up to 50% genetic link – but the behavioural and coping skills in those same families *also* account for up to 50%[21] [22]. So given a new foundation for

---

[23] National Centre for Eating Disorders: Information / Facts about Obesity.

[24] Set point: the weight range your body is biologically and genetically determined to weight. See also: Role of Set Point Theory in Regulation of Weight: R.B.Harris 1990

coping, different learning skills, your genetics do not *have* to become your destiny. Your biography however, could become your biology if the mindset – is, well, set. So why mention this at all?

It seems, and research is now backing this up[25], that the brain's response to certain forms of stimulus in certain individuals can be far more significant, so that what appears as lack of willpower, is in fact a far higher reaction, producing a need that increases in line with the criteria for substance addiction[26].

In addition to which, increased *availability* of that stimulus makes it a greater likelihood. So in an environment where highly tempting foods are so constantly available, and so constantly advertised, the possibility that those "cues" or promptings can trigger pathological responses is of great concern.

It IS however an area of immense interest and more recent research into the "neural correlates" of food addiction[25] confirm what I have long suspected: that we are not just a motley bunch of weak willed losers. I have had too many clients whose sustained effort and commitment just doesn't tally with that description – if anything, quite the *opposite*.

Working with hundreds of obese people over the years, my (uncollated) observations are that to some extent, this propensity probably exists at a *base* level in many people whose overeating is a continual issue. More often than not however, sufficient containment of an overeating habit *can* be achieved with the kind of recognition of other contributing factors provided in this book.

For the few, however, there seems to be a far greater struggle: if having taken on board lifestyle, physical activity and varying emotional triggers this struggle continues, then I suspect the above may be highly relevant. Finding ways to avoid anything which sets off cravings, (on every level but perhaps most notably again, crave inducing foods as mentioned earlier,) may not be an option.

---

[25] Neural Correlates of Food Addiction: Ashley N. Gearhardt et al (see appendix) Jama Psychiatry – formerly Archives of General Psychiatry Volume 68 No 8 August 2011.

[26] The Yale Food Addiction Scale (YFAS).

Most of us already know that given a significant emotional *event,* or set of events over time, the ability to hold back from an overeating reaction becomes far more difficult. There is also a link between a tendency to excessive carbohydrate consumption and insulin sensitivity[27]. Ditto sugar addiction which has a similar effect in similar areas of the brain as those used in substance abuse[28].

IF you are conscious of having an addictive side to you, this entire book will hopefully be of help, but in essence the core message will always be: DON'T GO THERE!! I may use humour but am entirely serious. Since I began working with obesity I have often been asked how I resist my own "solace for all seasons" – bread and butter. Since one slice rarely stops till the loaf is done – and some, here's how it goes: bread doesn't get brought into my home. If others have it, it gets eaten by them, and any remaining after guests have gone is disposed of. Sounds obsessive? You bet, but I am serious and it works for me and I do indulge socially, where pride usually prevents me from public gluttony! Of course this gets more difficult the more people you have living with you who you can hardly ban from everyday staple foods, but again, more of the how to deal with it – later.

---

[27] The X Factor Diet: For Lasting Weight Loss and Vital Health by Lesley Kenton Vermilion London 01/2005.
[28] "Sweet poison: why sugar is ruining our health" The Telegraph /Victoria Lambert 09/01/2014.

CULTURAL - ROLES:

How we see ourselves and unconsciously held beliefs and assumptions:
I refer to this in a later chapter - but our identity and how we see ourselves within the wider community belongs firmly in the Social Spectrum. I have only used three examples for the moment to flag this up but hopefully you will get the idea.

THE MOTHERLY IMAGE:
Even women who never had a weight problem until they had a baby can find themselves several stone up several years later. It starts with hormone changes and feeding for two... and while many manage to get their previous weight back after the first pregnancy, future additions to the family see not merely a repeat of the same process but having to cook different meals at different times. Yes your body goes through a physical change but not nearly to the same extent as your mind changes over the years. Realising you are suddenly grazing through the day or eating at each and every meal....can be a revelation in itself. Finding ways of not doing this will be where you have your work cut out... but the first step, as always, is catching yourself in action. Red handed at the fridge... etc!

THE GOOD HOST/ESS; THE GOOD GUEST:
Most of us when cooking for others want to offer food that is not just delicious, but plentiful. Having ample fare is part of being a good host. By the same token the "great" guest will be the one who asks for seconds, clearly showing enjoyment and thereby complementing the host. But are we buying into something which is no longer relevant?

Many people now dread yet another occasion which presents challenges for the overweight and already obese. Might it not be that the "good host" is now someone who takes time and effort to organize something less lethal than fries and "death by chocolate", especially in the work place which adds concerningly to comfort eating in the home.

Similarly, many yo-yo dieters find attempts at moderation once they achieve a weight they are happy with, are undermined by the presence of a multitude of treats in the house for visitors, should they pass by.

The issue is one of believing ourselves to be less than worthy as a host or mother or aunt if we do not have this to hand. Whilst this held true, more than true, in times of want, might this not be entirely redundant at the present time? Surely our concept of a good host should be someone that caters for our needs, and currently that is quite the opposite to being force fed cake and biscuits…?? Evidently food for thought!

How often do you have extra food in case friends or family visit?

-

Do you tend to cook just the right amount, or have an abundance for guests that gets left over?

-

How would you feel having just enough?

-

Would it make you anxious?

-

How much extra do you feel you need to provide to not feel anxious?

-

Would you worry what others might think?

-

As a guest, what might you prefer:
At work do's and professional meetings?

-

At social or family gatherings?

-

Make a list of your most recent examples.

-

-

THE GOOD WIFE versus NEW WOMAN!

A very independent, very ballsy client of mine finally shed the stones and maintained this, till she married. Two years later she returned to my door, mortified, weight gained, and some. Whilst looking back at where things had turned for the worse, she remembered her mother always saying "a good wife feeds her husband three good meals a day!" as would "any Northern lass". The problem was that she was not merely feeding the lucky man three good meals and more, but was darned if she would opt for ladylike, smaller portions, and to boot could match his drinking anytime. Realising what had been at play didn't mean the problem would vanish or that it would suddenly be a walk on the beach avoiding temptation, but it did flag up that her desire to stay slim was at odds with her need to match her husband's intake!

Add any examples of your own...

-

-

-

-

-

-

-

-

-

-

"Am I really hungry?"

"Will I be pleased with my choice in two hours time?"

THE BIGGER PICTURE and FILLING IN THE BACKDROP:

The purpose of the Social spectrum is to know increasingly, at any point, what is impacting your eating behaviours at any given time in the future, as well as the here and the now. Filling in the bigger backdrop takes on board the wider environment and a wider timescale.

The wider environment may be your living in a large town awash with terrific food outlets, meaning you run the gauntlet every time you leave home. It might be the proximity of extended family, making food centred visits a more frequent and difficult to avoid occurrence! The fuller picture here shows at a glance, everything which potentially disrupts your best laid eating plans and which you need to account for.

The wider timescale means you will be able to have an overview of your entire year, at any time.

The Rolling Event Calendar which you'll see later on enables an eight to twelve week overview, but taking on board your entire year puts you ahead of the fact and less likely to get caught short. It's no different to driving responsibly: we're alert to the road a hundred yards ahead as well as the cars directly in front and directly behind.

Most of us have times of the year which make weight holding easy or challenging depending on home or family commitments, changing seasons, extended holidays and so on.

For example:

- Extra cooking and the presence of children's snacks can present far more ongoing temptation during the school holidays.

- Professionally, there are often peak times of the year during which prolonged stress can play havoc with your eating behaviours.

- If your birthday's in say, January, and your nearest and dearest range from November through to March, taking you neatly to Easter, that's one long stretch of continued opportunity to over indulge, and at some point the "in for a penny in for a pound" mindset is likely to kick in…

- Anyone fortunate enough to have extended "holidays" can find their eating and drinking also in extended holiday mode. Unless you stick to set eating times and have perfect portion control, alarm bells should be ringing!

- Seasonally, many people find they are more likely to eat for comfort in the colder weather, while others find summer temptation with its outside barbeques and cocktails more difficult to resist.

Tip: Factor it in...

A fundamental error following weight loss is assuming the now virtuous mindset will last forever and immunise you against old habits and situations which still exist.

Most weight gain begins slowly enough till a tipping point ups the velocity and the exponential eating fest begins in earnest....

Your best immunity is to factor them in and if particular times are too challenging, work around them by "balancing the books" and reducing your weight ahead of the difficult time. I call this *paying it forward.*

PAYING IT FORWARD and going with the flow...

Going with the flow – don't push the river...

We all have times when we suddenly get a surge of energy to do tasks that we'd put off with a sinking heart for days or months. It's the same with dieting. Looking back over your weight patterns, you may find there's a time of year when your eating moderates or holds steadier than at other times. This is what we're looking for.

The principle behind *paying it forward* is that once you get the hang of it, it gives us brownie points ahead of time. It's an investment ahead of the fact.

Paying it forward for most people is easier as well as more exciting because instead of clearing up a mess that you're feeling upset and bad about, you're clearing up ahead of time and feeling virtuous instead.

Rather like Tai Chi, it's *going with the flow* of our energy.

Paying it forward ahead of holidays for example, means you're using the incentive as leverage. At worst you come back no heavier than you were before your weight loss and sometimes pride in achievement actually means you're just a tad more mindful of the usual holiday indulgence.

Paying it forward ahead of more challenging periods means you have one stress factor less to contend with, and are not spiralling up the scales with progressive years.

What it *averts* is the upset which catapults the best of us into an All or Nothing eating pattern which is hell bent on self destruct.

What it *provides* is a good safety net and room for movement.

What it *inspires* is indeed a feeling of greater safety and more meaningfully a positive mindset. Remember, it's much harder to motivate yourself once the incentive is gone.

Tip: "Return to base" on days "off"...

Going into treat mode for extended periods slides all too predictably into "give up" mode or total denial. Your easily visible Rolling Event Calendar means you can highlight the days when there is no social commitment or at least less to distract, and use these instead to "Return to Base"!

Tip: Staying on the safe side...

Returning to "base" on your days off... may only save a pound or so, but those few pounds make all the difference between throwing in the towel or being able to hold yourself back from the brink. It's that mindset matrix: past a certain point of weight gain, there's something of a more than the sum of the parts brain change! Keep within the safety net!

Tip: Nifty footwork...

It is very like a boxer or a footballer doing nifty footwork practise, jumping back to "Position One" with increasing ease but the more you practise, the easier it gets.

Even if you do not celebrate the predominant religious holidays, you may still be susceptible to national food advertising which ups the tempo with a vengeance from November 1st each year, bringing a smorgasbord of culinary delights straight off the screen and into your living room, along with a tempting array of extra goodies in all the shops and in offices.

Tip: TV ads on mute...

People often underestimate the power of advertising and the effect of the visual on our senses, but underestimate at your peril! Get into the habit of clicking the mute button during the TV ads and direct your focus elsewhere! You don't have to be an overeater to buy into the seasonal "entitlement factor", (I'll treat myself as it's Easter / Christmas etc...) and you can practically *taste* those ads!

Using your Eating Behaviour Blueprint... be brutally honest...

By now your Eating Behaviour Blueprint will already be giving you invaluable information but you will still need to use it as objectively as you are able, and be brutally honest with yourself about how you operate:

I don't want anyone to feel bad. It serves nothing. Feeling bad or guilty simply acts as a trigger half the time for reactive eating. It's about taking a good hard look at your eating behaviours to see how you can best work at any given time. Looking at your weight fluctuation over a wider time scale enables better decision making about when you most easily take action, and when it's best to ease up.

If your tendency is to put off the inevitable, pretending that you can "balance the books" at a different time will however, up the pressure and up the likelihood of an increasingly crazed eating response! Notice where you kid yourself!

You *cannot* afford to delude yourself if there won't be an easier time, nor can you afford to let yourself off when it comes to "paying it back."

Especially once your emotional eating behaviours are brought into the equation you will recognise there will always be times, sometimes horribly prolonged, where you struggle and feel no headway is being made or worse, that you are sliding all the way back to square one.

The good news is your heightened awareness means you can't ever go back to square one. It's not a revolving door but a spiralling staircase, so that every return to a familiar "lesson" has a better perspective each time, and with it new information.

Moreover, when we struggle it can only be because we have our eyes wide open and our awareness is far higher. Denial knows no struggle till after the event. The going can get tough, but that's only because you've already come a long way.

So take heart!

What will happen over the years is that some of your eating habits will drop off easily, while others are a work in progress. Knowing the difference will make life easier as well as giving you fantastic confidence at what you have managed successfully.

Paying it forward in action...
Look to when your weight, and hence your eating habits, more naturally moderates during the year and use this as your bench mark. Past experience as well as your weight history will help back this up.

Weighing yourself and keeping a record:
Because recurrent weight gain is mostly a direct result of doing whatever we did before, it's a really good idea to keep a weekly weight diary of some kind to keep on track which means... you'd be best to weigh yourself at least once a week.

Even if thinking back you can't remember what happened with your eating, a slow or sudden incline in weight gain on particular dates gives enough information for you to be on the alert. It's part of that evidence collecting detective work which enables you, at some point, to review your year and make better decisions on that basis.

Looking at the events you already have penned in, including national and personal holidays, highlight whenever it would seem more easy for you to moderate your eating in advance.

When might some of those dates or times be?

When would your schedule most allow for time to focus on yourself?

When would there be more calm, less stress and less temptation around?

Make a note of as many "windows of opportunity" as you can, and think back too to when this has happened most naturally in the past.

-

-

-

-

-

If there's little to no evidence of moderation and the word is practically off your radar, reflect on what for you is usually a more stable time of year, even by degree. Find even the tiniest foot hold to begin. If this is you and you are so worn out with yourself you feel little but exasperation and disappointment, imagine for a moment that the person valiantly searching for just a tiny way in is a much loved friend. You would have nothing but compassion and love and admiration for this friend's continual perseverance. Please, please, have this for yourself because it is this quality of caring which will get you furthest. Whatever the outcome.

Overview...

Putting together your past experience, the information from your Social Spectrum, and your year ahead, when do you believe you have the best chance of beginning and maintaining a diet, if this is your intention?

-

-

-

When might the odds be more against a new start, or put another way, when do you notice you most easily put on weight during the year?

-

-

-

When might you most need to *pay it forward?*

-

-

When could you most easily *pay it forward?*

-

-

Maintaining an ongoing vigilance and staying mindful might seem an awful lot of effort for the long term but again it's like driving: a lot becomes automatic but your eyes are still open - you don't take a nap on the motorway. You will "stop and park" occasionally, but you'll have planned it into the broad sweep of your year. You will have become accountable for your eating behaviours as much as you are accountable for safe driving or keeping to commitments. We don't think "oh heck, I've gotta do that for*ever!*" - if it's halfway important we just take it for granted. Any argument in our heads when something isn't settled in our minds is a drain on reserves and adds subtly but indisputably to any emotional eating. It's like we have a cup of resilience that is either refreshed or diminished. Indecision wears down and diminishes. A settled decision refills. Once it's accepted as a necessary there isn't the same conflict. We get on with it. This is what needs to happen with planning our eating ahead of time.

* * *

Another necessary aspect of the bigger picture are life cycles and transitions.

While their impact ranges from the subtle to the dramatic, the affect on our lives can last years and create an emotional "tipping point" which makes sense of reactive overeating we can't otherwise explain. If something we accept as normal is actually a long term source of upset, it takes little to understand the knock on effect making us susceptible in areas we might otherwise handle well enough.

Our roles and how we see ourselves and whether we afford them value (or not) have to be considered in that wider perspective.

If there's conflict between who we are and how we are living we might get on with it, but even the greatest pragmatist may have a chronic level of discontent chip chipping just below the surface and wearing them down. That cup of resilience can end up on permanent "low reserve" without our realising why! Insight, at the least, enables greater compassion in understanding our eating behaviours. Compassion can lessen some of the negative reaction, and understanding gives us choice where we may have felt there was none. Let's have a look at some of those rites of passage.

LIFE CYCLES and TRANSITIONS

"Who am I?

What is my name?

Where are the sandwiches?"

(someone from the Findhorn community in North West Scotland!)

The social and the emotional are of course always inextricably interwoven since what we do effects how we feel, which in turn affects what we decide to do, the spin off playing havoc with or moderating our eating patterns and behaviours and so on and so forth...

Rarely is the social infrastructure more imbued with intense emotion than with some of our major life transitions. It is for this reason I have placed it here, between the two, with its ever constant two way ripple literally impacting the balance of the scales!

Life cycles are invariably Rites of Passage[29], and even when we anticipate a positive "rite of passage", such as turning 21, the birth of a child, a new career, it brings in its wake a transformation of some kind, however subtle: how we see ourselves and unconsciously held values and beliefs, our place in society, what we do with ourselves, our roles, whether we are stuck in them or regret their passing, all provide a framework for emotional eating.

Whilst celebration and contentment go hand in hand all too easily

---

[29] Erik Erikson: Stages of Psychosocial Development.

with indulgence and ensuing weight gain, I have chosen to focus on the challenging changes: reactive eating is never so much in evidence as when we are using food as a default position in face of the unknown. Feeding ourselves, and I mean overfeeding here as opposed to balanced nourishment, feels familiar, and if we keep eating we hold to the familiar in otherwise alien territory. Insight at least is a first port in the storm. What we do with that insight comes later.

EMPTY NEST SYNDROME / BEREAVEMENT / BROKEN DREAMS / REGRET: The Void versus The Good Life...

It's often said that when one door closes, another opens. Platitudes apart, the thing with life transitions, especially if it's the ending of a whole era that's meant a lot to you and has been a valuable part of who you are, your history and your identity, is that there's often an overly long bit in the middle where we wonder "WHO AM I *NOW*?". "WHO AM I and what is my worth now that my contribution to my family or the world is over??" Now that I am no longer an active mum or someone's partner or working?? WHO AM I NOW if I can't have children? No longer sexually active / attractive / old etc etc. That "middle" bit can prolong itself uncomfortably over some years at times until we have adjusted. And past that first 3 to 6 months when endorphins as well as matters of practicality serve to protect, the early period of mourning can leave in its wake a huge void.

There are many types of mourning, many dreams left broken and unrealised. Whilst there are accepted transitions, and sometimes rites of passage where a ritual might accompany the passing of a stage, (divorce, retirement, bereavement and accompanying anniversaries), equally there are many less visible passings: the erosion of good health and bodily functions with all we once took for granted and with it loss of autonomy; couples who separate without having married or had children may often receive far less in the way of support or sympathy – lack of officialdom in this respect whilst averting the entanglements of divorce, extracting dividend after the fact for this lack of bureaucratic recognition. There is by default, an absence of validation, nothing that bears witness to something deeply felt and meaningful. Most poignantly perhaps, the death of a child, or women and their partners who have experienced still births or miscarriages who come through with emptiness instead of a child.

The death of long loved pets too, can be deeply mourned but don't quite fit the mould in terms of the usual sympathy and support: careers which haven't worked out; exams not passed... Especially too in the absence of the wider family, the sense of "who the hell am I and what on earth am I doing" can leave quite a vacuum all too easily filled with comfort eating to fill the existential gap... or whatever emotion has surfaced, and keeps surfacing. Added to which of course, is a *literal* gap of *time* during the days or nights, as well as the more emotional gap of our function, and what we *did* or had expected to do with that time. Even for people who are ready for their new life, or for the more welcome change that a transition has brought upon them, this can be especially visible as weight is gained through an increase in social or daytime eating. Moving from the constraints of a life with too much to do to one where we do not yet know what to do with the time, is rather like moving to an eternally long weekend.

For all of this, finding a new focus to revitalize you, to give meaning to your life, is probably going to be one of the best ways to ensure you are not simply overeating to comfort yourself, or because you are at a loss as to what to do and how to be. It's also immensely important to have given time to honour and acknowledge whoever or whatever has been lost or never even realised in the first place. Blocking out with an array of practical time fillers will go so far, and is often initially as necessary as it is cathartic, but there is something about stages of mourning and bereavement that are pretty compelling and not easily sat on without cost.[30] [31] We seek often to move on as quickly as possible to escape pain and discomfort, yet this is rarely fully possible till we allow space and time to sit with where we're at. Eating as an emotional reaction – as I look at in the next chapter, is your clearest sign that something in you really does need nourishment and attention, but of a different kind.

---

[30] www.recover-from-grief.com/7stages-of-grief

[31] Elisabeth Kubler-Ross: Death: The Final Stage of Growth 1975

Reactive Eating and the Emotional Spectrum: What Lies Beneath?

It is understood that energy can be transformed, but never wasted or destroyed[32].

Maladaptive patterns may arise to maintain homeostasis, to stay the same way of being, but there is still a function within this that makes logical sense.

If the red warning light in your car, computer, any machine you value, began flashing, you would hardly imagine that taking a hammer and smashing it would make the problem go away.

When you feel you can't stop eating, binging, nibbling, you might feel pathetic, useless, or whatever array of words you choose to ascribe yourself...

... but your body / mind is not stupid or pathetic... it is doing something for a reason.

It has a FUNCTION...

- Reading through the pages, which of the reasons do you most relate to?
- What is your body saying?
- If your body could speak, what would the dialogue be? How would that conversation be going..?

---

[32] A philosophical leap from one of Richard Feynman's Lectures on Physics: Conservation of Energy

WHAT LIES BENEATH: THE EMOTIONAL SPECTRUM
"Am I really hungry?"

How often do you raid the larder, the biscuit packet, the fridge… at the slightest hint of a problem, without even being hungry or stopping to question why you are doing it or what you are feeling?

Using food or drink as a reaction to emotion is what usually puts all your weight holding efforts on a possible train to nowhere. You keep coming back to the same place.

Assuming, for the moment, you've factored your new diet into the day, that you've planned what you will eat and not get caught short, any failure to stay your ground is less likely to be lack of resolve but the intensity of an emotion seeking its usual opiate. It's often the one thing we haven't planned around, let alone reckon on its strength.

Emotions can be upsetting and turbulent as much as others create pleasure and excitement. They also provide information:

YOUR BODY as MESSENGER!!
We can feel deeply disappointed and call ourselves useless, weak willed, pathetic, any number of self berating adjectives but in fact our **CRAVINGS HAVE A FUNCTION: they are telling us something! PROVIDING INFORMATION!! Your mind and body are not pathetic but doing something for a REASON!**

RED WARNING LIGHTS
If the red warning light or whatever you have on your car dashboard began flashing, you would hardly get a hammer and smash it, thinking "there, that's solved that stupid problem!". You would be aware that something was wrong and begin looking in order to repair it. Your eating behaviours are no different. To the extent that some aspect of our nourishment is missing, (I hasten to add this could equally be physical if we are deplete in some way), to the extent that there is some imbalance in our lives or our bodies, we look elsewhere to lessen the tension that arises as a result. We seek, instinctively, to redress the balance and to compensate. One of those compensators is food and drink.

LEARNING TO READ THE SIGNALS

Maladaptive patterns may arise to maintain a particular way of being, (homeostasis) and these patterns may eventually be to our cost, but perversely, we *are* doing the best we can at any given moment.

We *do,* however, need to pay attention to the warning light, which is our eating behaviour: becoming aware of the emotions that prompt overeating will give some idea as to where they stem and so what to do instead. It may not always be possible, but it is a pointer in the right direction.

If you have covered an emotion with eating for so long you barely recognize what it relates to, take note then of any situations, as in who and what and where, which surround it or precipitate it. And have patience... things won't necessarily reveal themselves by demand, but gentle observation is already turning a leaf. Again, do keep a record, and date it. When people ask what can they do to start changing things, that *is* one hundred per cent your first step. Observation and "collecting the evidence" *is* your first step. Remember, *recognition* is key to success. You have already begun.

So here are a range of *emotionally driven reasons* which run the gamut from the everyday, simple, mundane, to the more complex. As I have gone into more depth than in previous chapters, you may prefer to scan through initially and see what grabs your attention. Returning later may give you pause for thought, and time to absorb more fully if something resonates. If it does, notice what leaps to mind. Notice whether there is an immediate *feeling or thought or physical sensation* of any kind. Notice too if comes *wrapped inside a memory.* As before make a note *of* it. We'll take it from there later.

COMFORT EATING

I've begun with this as most overeating will have a comfort factor of some kind: whether it just tastes great and gives into temptation, whether it's to pass time, whether it's to alleviate or block out a negative emotion, or even whether it's succumbing to an unknown compulsion: the initial sense is one of relief or comfort, even if simply by virtue of reducing the tension, however transitory, and even if hours later we are regretting the indulgence.

"There there, have a biscuit and it will be better" syndrome, often starts when we are small and have hurt ourselves or are upset and need comforting in some way. Eating for comfort and to feel better is instilled early on and maintained to perfection through adulthood: we feel upset or wanting in some way and look for comfort... Eating to help ourselves feel better is an easy reaction, but it is still none the less *reactive.* On a positive level it's an enjoyable form of "self nurturing", but if it goes unchecked or you simply can't stop, then it's happening at a cost and you might want to question whether it's self nurturing, or self harming.

MOOD ALTERING
The most obvious comfort is that however briefly, our mood is altered. At its most basic, if we enjoy what we eat, it's very easy to go for another helping... not because we are still hungry - but because it made us feel good. It altered our mood for the better, even if "better" is a case of blocking out a more negative emotion. If the feel good factor is indeed utterly fantastic, you might want to weigh up the pounds and ask "Will I be pleased with my choice in two hours time?" while considering where you might need nourishment in other ways in your life... If, at worst, the overeating is so extreme and habit driven that you no longer actually experience hunger let alone a feel good factor, the need to explore what lies beneath will be crucial. Turning the focus of attention away from the calories to whatever it is that creates the eating demand... for the meantime at least, is categorically the first step. It doesn't mean you have to fully resolve the emotional source of your reactive eating, which might simply add yet another layer of stress into the equation. What it does mean is that you acknowledge what is happening and take it from there. Often the acknowledgement in its own right has a softening effect on a compulsion. If your eating behaviour is taking centre stage, and seems therefore – attention seeking, maybe it's because it really does require your attention! No mystery there! But the approach must be as it would a screaming or abandoned child: gently but firmly, and with love.

167

ALERT!

Noticing whether your need for comfort or need to eat for any reason when you're not actually physically hungry, is mild, moderate, or intensely compulsive, is especially important in detecting which of the following emotions or situations are driving the eating behaviours.

CONTENTMENT

No prize winning here once you've read through the rest for noticing this is the odd one out: in each and every other emotion, the food is used either as a coping mechanism or to fill a gap. For some people, harmony in their world means their eating becomes less erratic and naturally moderates. One lady some years ago described how she had overeaten for years, till subsequent to a divorce, she rented a houseboat for a year.

Who knows whether the divorce or living a life she loved contributed more greatly to her naturally moderating food intake but suffice that her eating simply curbed – almost of its own volition. Conversely many people describe their eating increasing when they are very happy and very settled. Sceptic that I am, and taking to task the warning light analogy, I occasionally question whether there is not the tiniest bit of boredom in such apparent bliss, and a tendency therefore to fill this yet again with eating as a time filler. This may of course not be the case, but it's worth checking sooner rather later whether a different distraction might serve better for the long term!

STRESS

"The extent to which we perceive the external locus of control to be greater than our internal locus of control..."

In a way, the *distress* from which this comes could be placed anywhere and everywhere along both the social and emotionally driven spectrums.

Thinking back too, to the swinging metal balls and their *chain reaction,* stress is one of those frequent tipping points: trace its roots backwards, far enough, and we discover the source, the true issue from which it emanates. Cast our line of vision forward, and the far flung shadow of its disturbing effects becomes all too clear.

As with any emotion, the shift in stress related eating patterns might be subtle enough to go unnoticed, which is why a change in your weight as well as rising anxiety, can be a more useful indicator in pinpointing when something begins to get out of hand: as the definition suggests however, it's all about perception, and the issue is our felt sense of having enough control. It's highly subjective, and what one person feels they need to restore the status quo will be very different from another. The "status quo" for the record, being whatever restores a person's sense of control, and hence their internal emotional balance. In the case of Sally, who I mention in a later chapter, washing the dishes restored the balance! Of course within and beneath that stress will lie other emotions, but to get to the root from a practical perspective, we need to follow it back to its starting place.

Tracing the roots...
There are many factors[33], but most of them will come down in some way or other to 5 main areas:

Relationships: Family / Partnerships / Children / Social
Finances
Work
Health
Home / Domestic

It is rarely necessary to completely eradicate the cause of something any more than it would be possible, but it will always be necessary to address it *enough*. Most of us, given a calm enough environment, can get on with our lives, but there's always a straw that breaks the camel's back, with its domino effect on our eating and drinking behaviours. Since too, we are often so busy that unless an issue becomes top priority we park it to the side, excessive weight gain is the warning light that brings it back off the back burner into the must do now pile.

---

[33] For example The Holmes & Rahe Stress Scale 1967

Area of Origin	Stress levels	Behaviour (your clue)	Outcome
Work	normal	eating	Weight gain /
Finances	manageable	behaviour	Weight loss
Health	considerable	drinking /	
Relationship	high	smoking / other	
Family / children			
Home (i.e. where you live /changes in the home etc)			

Case example...

Mandy had successfully lost about four stone when she began having work done on her bathroom, kitchen and living room. She'd chosen to have the lot done in one go to get it over and done with, but it was taking far longer than expected and was far more unsettling than she could have imagined: apart from not being able to cook, there were disagreements with the builders on a daily basis, and she felt constantly tense and with "nowhere to hide". Within a fortnight her old "crisps and pizza" habit had re-emerged with a vengeance, her weight was back on the up, and she felt desperate. Mandy felt additionally upset at her inability to stay calm on the basis that, while very intrusive, it was hardly "a crisis."

Although Mandy was right in it not actually being a crisis, I pointed out that many of us react similarly with this all too familiar scenario (I for one!). Further, there were a couple of exacerbating factors adding to the upset, but I'll return to that when we look at the effect of high risk combinations in tipping us over the edge... (Putting it All Together).

The upset at being upset scenario...

Put into perspective, Mandy said for the most part she could tolerate the tension, but what really sent her into a spin was feeling unable to control the resulting eating behaviour, and her weight paying the price. *That...* was where her stress levels actually peaked.

Asked what one thing could help her feel better and less upset, she said just having some private space to herself and being able to cook might do the trick, and wondered whether she might perhaps move into her bedroom for the duration, making it a kind of temporary studio until she had her house back.

In the event she also remembered she had a little Belling oven cooker and hob which she'd bought for a caravan in the past, so along with her microwave and a make shift table, she got busy that evening converting her new "bed sit". When Mandy returned the following week I knew the instant I saw her face it had worked!

... one small change...

Not everything will be so easily remedied, but there is usually **something** we can do to temper the upset and lower the stress that leads to bad eating habits. A lot of the time we can't change the fundamentals of a situation, but we might be able to get creative with the tipping point or reduce the straw that breaks the camel's back. Mandy's was need for private space and being able to cook.

Make a list of your most frequent stress inducing situations.

-

-

-

-

-

Ask yourself:

In a situation that is causing you stress, what is the bit that tips it over the edge?

-

-

-

Tip: If you're unsure - your eating behaviour will usually be the clue! Notice when it slots into action!

Ask yourself:

*What do you believe you most **need** to feel ok enough?*

-

*What **can** you change, or do, that might enable this?*

-

Tip: You will know very quickly if you have hit the button either by simply imagining it, or as soon as you begin to put it into action. Lowering of stress levels are very quickly apparent!

UPSET / SADNESS / GRIEF... Feeling hurt, sad, alone even if not lonely, neglected, abandoned, isolated, unloved or unlovable, feeling foolish, uncertain, lacking in confidence etc... (See also Life Cycles and Transitions)

As with comfort eating, earlier, using food to console, make better etc: at times the emotion we seek to appease may be obvious, especially if the cause is recent. Sometimes though we are oblivious to the habit, however obvious you'd expect it to be. If the feeling is a longstanding one, we may no longer recall why or how it began, let alone its link to our eating behaviour. The purpose in tracing its roots and discovering the link is solely to address it sufficiently. We can do the diet, lose the weight etc, but to the extent that some eating behaviours are a way of coping with an emotion still with us from a past or current event, it is highly likely the behaviour will reassert itself until it is genuinely let go of, enough, for our peace of mind to resume. This is absolutely not about digging up things which are dead and buried and should remain so. It's about having the courage to look at stuff which is still jostling around in the attic or banging on the door of the cellar!! Here's the clue: if you have a heightened emotional reaction to the thought or mention of something, however much in the past, it is very likely in the box marked "still in the present." Otherwise it couldn't evoke the same intensity of emotion. If something is no longer relevant – there is far less emotion present, and certainly not on a daily basis. Which means it won't be driving your eating behaviour.

Be mindful that bereavement can trigger anger as well as grief, which might get "buried" simply because it is a less obviously acceptable emotion to deal with at the time. Added to this, intense feelings can get put to the side simply through fear that we will be overwhelmed and not be able to cope[34]. As much with our daily lives and the need to keep functioning, as the feelings themselves. In light of this, again, take heart that a *gentle* approach works wonders. No one needs to be a hero or put their head in the lion's mouth! Gently as well as less, is often more.

COMPENSATORY CONTROL & PROCRASTINATION

On a general level, and as further described below, overeating may have been a way of replacing something you're stuck with, or can't have in the moment, (and at some points in your life that might be "a moment" of several years…) with something you *can* have, or can do, immediately and in the here and now.

Similarly, putting things off can cast a long shadow into the future.

Be open to discover, should you not already know, what it is you are attempting to control or defer. And why? Whether it is through fear of failure or tedium, and even whether the concern is justified. It may need a reality check. If procrastination is the issue, how long has your life been on hold? I have to raise my hand here and confess the completion of this book has been an extortionate time in the coming. If areas of your life are suffering and your weight is soaring, there's a do or die point at which it is no longer acceptable. Have a look at the monkey story later on and see whether you can do a u-turn.

---

[34] Living with Death and Dying – Elisabeth Kubler-Ross 1997 Scribener
Working it Through: An Elisabeth Kubler-Ross Workshop on Life, Death and Transitions. Simon & Schulster 1981.

BOREDOM

I've gone into this one in greater depth because, as with the need for comfort, the need to eat rather than find ourselves bored is almost a gap filling activity par excellence. People may not always realise they "do" boredom so frequently, but if you're a finger tapping adrenalin junkie with an even moderate stress level, you could be in here somewhere!

Oversimplifying once again to make the point – there's mundane, everyday, commonplace boredom, and there's the more prolonged, what I call core level, life issue kind of boredom... and the first... is likely to be exacerbated by the second:

MUNDANE BOREDOM

Very useful to look at what to you means boredom: a teenager might be bored with "nothing to do" and an inability to keep themselves occupied and entertained. A mature person by contrast might be "bored" because they are stuck doing something they'd rather not be doing, i.e. tax forms, housework, mundane tasks etc, and eating defers the inevitable. Again a form of *procrastination.*

It's easy too, to feel "bored" in the evenings when we might rather be doing something other than eating in front of the TV, but feel too jaded to do it.

Whichever, there's an inherent anxiety in boredom, and people will expend considerable effort to prevent or remedy it. Hence we will often eat to "fill a gap" rather than from genuine hunger.

Begin to notice what you were doing when you went for that snack, if you weren't actually hungry, and when...

List down what it is you are stuck with at the moment, or putting off. Or what you would rather be doing if you had the energy, more get up and go?

-

-

-

-

PROLONGED, OR EXISTENTIAL BOREDOM
Also covering *Looking for Satisfaction; Frustration* etc:

Similar to, but more deeply felt and prolonged over time than above.

If you are dissatisfied with your life, perhaps constantly occupying yourself with other people's needs, or simply stuck in a very deep, over familiar rut... You may equally succumb to "filling the gap" and "satisfying yourself" with food.

Where would you rather *be*? What would you rather be *doing*? Whether this is an extreme situation, or the reality, to a given extent, of some aspect of your daily existence, addressing this enables you, at best, to resolve it, and at the least – to become more conscious of precisely *what function* is served by the overeating – and to make some change, however small. A mother with three young children *cannot* just get up and swan off, leastways not without serious consequence, but becoming conscious of what's happening begins to put her back in control, at her own driving wheel and the option of some let up. Most jobs or ways of being have an element of *something* we dislike, or find tedious. Can we rearrange it in some way? Often, if a situation has become chronic and entrenched, we might feel that only dramatic action will save the day when in reality, a small change will provide the release in pressure we are seeking: I know that several years into working more daily, regular hours as a counsellor with a business to run, the wanderlust for my previous life – not so much as cabin crew but for the fantastic travel it afforded, really began to kick in. Increasingly over the months I was not only overspending again, always a big clue with me... but beginning to fantasize about giving up altogether the business franchise I'd worked long and hard for, and doing my nomadic bit.... Thankfully I realised in time that I'd not taken a holiday for five years, and that the "wandering adventurer" in me needed honouring!! Dumbing it down was beginning to create a potentially irrevocable course of action and a volcanic eruption in the making: what seemed incredible at the time was the benefit of taking a fortnight away - my yearnings disappeared as did the increasing bouts of overspending: if ever there had been a clear indication as to the perils of the pressure cooker blowing or "talking myself out of" things which on the face of it seem trivial or frivolous – this was it.

Write down whatever it is you would rather be doing, even if it is highly impractical and off the radar with regard to your present way of life.

If wholly impractical, what might even remotely fill the need, other than eating?

Cast your mind through things that you love, that satiate you in some way, that engage your attention in a positive way. Boredom often arises because we have overridden doing anything heartfelt. We may see it as secondary to work or family, or feel it takes time or money we don't have. It may be though that doing something, even for ten or fifteen minutes a day, which restores a sense of heartfelt space or enjoyment, is no longer an option. Make a list ranging from the smallest potentially feasible, to your wildest heartfelt desire. (See Lighting your Fire chapter)

-

-

-

-

-

-

Again, it's initially more about acknowledgement and awareness than immediately putting something into effect. Unless of course, it is immediately doable!

AVOIDANCE (superficial / mundane...)

Feeling guilty about not doing things we "should" be doing and being "lazy"? That old chestnut "prolonged procrastination"?? Eating instead, and thus avoiding the task and "productively" engaging yourself – is often a seemingly wonderful way to replace things we don't especially want to do or can't quite muster the effort to start, with something nice we *can* immediately do in its place!! And we can convince ourselves that after all, we do need to eat, it's necessary for survival etc..! If you are using food in this way you may need to learn how to allow yourself free time. People need time to revitalise themselves. If you feel you have to be constantly productive to be worthy, this may be what you need to explore more, and ideally let go of in part, rather than "dieting" whenever you pile on the pounds. Conversely and more practically, you may need to re-evaluate how you organize your time. Schedule only what you can realistically manage in a day and let the rest go until tomorrow. Or begin experimenting with doing the least favoured chore at the outset of the day, and how that feels... meaning the rest of the day you're already on a winner..!! Finally if your back is really against the wall and the resistance, rational or otherwise, at having to get on with something fills you with dread, allowing yourself to tackle it for just 15 minutes, and no more, can ease the way in and turn procrastination and the time it wastes on its head. (See "The 15 minute Rule"[35])

Equally working out what you need to prioritize, what you can delegate, and what you might let go of can be a minimal but productive exercise in de-cluttering mental space and enabling a forward moving flow... without the need to forestall with eating! (See later on under Do, Delegate or Dump!)

AVOIDANCE (more complex, deeper level...)
INSULATION / ANAESTHETISING / NUMBING / BLOCKING OUT
anger / hurt etc...

Using food to stop emotional or physical pain. Eating as much or as fast as you can when others – such as parents when we're younger – are arguing or fighting around us – as if the food will somehow block the noise. As with stress factors, eating a lot can have a numbing quality. Excess food sitting in the stomach fermenting can create drowsiness, numbness, and a general loss of energy which helps to insulate the feelings and keep some of the pain at bay. This can become an entrenched reflex action over the years which may need additional resolve and clarity to lessen or undo. If

---

[35] Caroline Buchanan: The 15 Minute Rule – Right Way 2012.

its function in avoiding pain is effectively achieved, and the habit so longstanding you barely notice its existence, you will likely only be drawn to peel away the layers when something more ailing beckons: this may be a matter of your weight creating health issues, or simply the need to discover what blocked out memories are preventing a fuller way of living, if this happens to be the case.

Ask yourself *what it is that you are avoiding, or blocking out, or numbing by eating instead?*

-

-

-

Notice next time you eat at the onset of a negative feeling. What is the feeling? What is the situation that is triggering it? What are your thoughts? Are you aware of any physical tensions, such as holding your breath or breathing fast or shallow?

Simply noticing is all that is needed at first. Just gently tiptoeing to have a better look. No big moves!

AVOIDANCE and ANGER (stuffing / stuffing down…)

Particularly if you were taught as a child that anger is an inappropriate emotion, you might find that you use food to "stuff down" your anger, or irritation or upset. Sometimes a way of not having to communicate anything remotely uncomfortable which then becomes the accepted norm, other times a survival response to avoiding physically or emotionally abusive behaviour. This may not have been taught explicitly but simply, as with most things, by way of example. How your mum, dad, or whoever brought you up, behaved in this respect is the example we are most likely to have followed, or "swallowed whole", without question. A case of nurture impacting nature, it's not a question of good or bad but it can be a helluva job undoing a reaction that does its job at the cost of your weight and health.

Ask yourself *whenever you find this happens in the future:*

Do I know why I am angry, or what is making me feel angry?

-

-

-

Am I clear about what I would like to say, or is it a mix of an awful lot over a long time, with many added emotions?

-

-

-

What is it I would most like **to say?**

-

-

-

Who would I be saying it to?

-

-

What am I afraid might happen if I did speak my mind? What is the outcome I fear?

-

-

This is not a suggestion that you take the offensive... but rather an opportunity for you to notice the link between your anger and your eating. You may then want to check the reality of the situation... and whether any person concerned is even aware of how you feel. Assertiveness in essence is about clear communication, and often as not that starts with ourselves. Striking when the iron is cold, rather than hot, allows for temperatures to cool and reason to replace emotional reaction.

Additionally if your resistance has legitimate cause for concern, you may not want to add fuel to the fire! Leastways not without consideration.

Finally, if you do summon the courage to say something to whoever, whatever you do – **resist** the (often overwhelming) urge to tell them "you always / never…" etc. It is the most likely way of ending up with the very heated emotions and situation that makes you "eat your words" to begin with. It's a case of – keep calm, stay specific, and stay in the present time. (For more on clear communication, see the chapter How We See Things.)

REVENGE

Think about your situation. Who are you trying to get back at by overeating or by being overweight? Sometimes it's getting back at a parent who tried to dictate our eating habits throughout our upbringing, making our worthiness seem conditional upon our slimness, and "eating when and how I like" is our first step at real autonomy, proving our independence when we leave home. It may be a self destructive form of self expression but it's something over which another person cannot exert their control. The extra pounds are screaming out "You can't control my body!! You can't control what I do!!!"

The problem is you're in rather an ivory tower.

Other times it could be someone who has let us down or betrayed us, (or at least we believe this to be the case…) or a partner who makes clear they love us best when we are slim. By implication – becoming overweight or fat is a deal breaker. There can be a kind of underlying "You should love me however I am" syndrome at play here. Whatever… hugely understandable but again, any of these reactions come at a cost. There's a native American Indian saying: "When we get angry we give our power away to the other." No one suffers but ourselves!

Yet again however, we may not even realise our eating reaction is linked, so as with the emotions above, getting clear and upping the awareness is part of the process. You're not building Rome in a day. It's also important to know that awareness and insight alone don't always have an immediately corrective influence on a longstanding habit. If only! It may take a while for the emotion to lessen its tug on the impulse to eat, which could feel like a lasso pulling you in. You might need an intervention of some kind to steer you away from automatic eating behaviour. We'll be coming to that later on.

SHAME, GUILT and INSULATION
(See also Weight as a Barrier to Intimacy-3, further down.)

I've differentiated this from above... because the function of the insulation here is to cover an emotion that can be particularly self destructive: whilst shame and guilt *might* have a rational base, they can equally be a product of either upbringing or abusive occurrences and are particularly difficult to eradicate. Shame in particular tries to hide itself, (because we're ashamed of the shame...) and tends to pervade the very core of one's being. Even when parenting has been misguided rather than overtly bad, on some level – the child or young person maturing may deem themselves never quite good enough, fast enough, perfect enough, in sum, simply – not enough. Whatever they do may feel as though it falls short compared to the standards set explicitly or implicitly, and however much rationale shows this not to be the case, it still doesn't feel convincing. Where conversely the parenting, or a relationship, has been at fault and physically or verbally abusive, this is still frequently and poignantly carried by the person receiving harm as self shame. Events such as rape and assault can also be a shamefully carried secret and produce deep feelings of self loathing even when someone might have been far too young to stop it. Eating can be a coping mechanism that insulates the pain or buries intolerable negative emotion. The reaction to this is deep and corrosive, and whilst cognitive behavioural therapy (CBT) will be a useful starting point - my personal opinion and experience is that intellectual reasoning alone rarely cuts the head of the snake. Recognition that something needs to be done and that much is amiss may be an essential first step, but love and support and compassion will be integral to self healing in whatever way is possible.

Overeating here and its function of insulating and blocking out the shame which in itself is deeply painful, can almost feel like a survival instinct.

One of my clients would reduce her overeating and slim down with relative ease, till she neared the weight she'd been when as a teenager, she'd been badly traumatised. While she realised that the risk of attracting a repeat occurrence was highly unlikely, keeping weight on hid her femininity and her reverting to overeating in order to regain the weight felt to her like she was doing it to survive. It was an instinctive reaction to an alarm signal from the body. It is often said our biography becomes our biology and our bodies hold our memories. In every way, the sum total of our lives affects our level of inner wellbeing, and ease, or dis-ease. Whether that dis-ease impacts us mentally, emotionally, or more physically will depend on our make up and our predisposition. It's not a mystery or rocket science, just nature doing what it does.

Because of this, work with the body and with the breath is especially cathartic in enabling release of trapped emotional pain. It probably won't happen overnight, but along with talking to someone professional, can really help ease the pain out of where it might be stuck, splinter like, in our system.

Forms of chanting, work with the body, hatha yoga including pranayama which is working with the breath, Alexander Technique, dance, Gabriel Roth 5 Rhythms, Biodanza, in **conjunction with** Cognitive Behavioural Therapy or one of the talking therapies can be immensely useful. Lest you think that all sounds a bit too "out there" ... working with sound, indeed just singing, opens the diaphragm. When we have become emotionally closed, we tend to breathe more shallowly. The diaphragm is sometimes referred to as the gate to the unconscious, since when opened fully and regularly it can evoke recollection and a release of stuck emotions.

Which means if you suspect there's a lot of buried emotion covered by your eating you may do well to enlist professional support. If you think about divers going into the depths, they never, never go alone.

On a lighter note, singing in itself does a lot of the soul lifting... but chanting kind of digs deeper. Whether joining a choir (The Rock Choir, now all over UK, accepts *anyone!!*) or something more overtly spiritual, (gospel, church, bhajans...) it helps the diaphragm and the lungs to open, and it brings joy!

More currently, Eye Movement Desensitization Remedy (EMDR)[36] and Somatic Experiencing Therapy[37] are used as a way of releasing past trauma which has become trapped, rather like shell shock, in the emotional part of our brain. Fight or flight has long since worked its way into common parlance but less considered is the "freeze" bit, which is where emotional memory slots into the limbic area, designed to pop up and "warn" if something similar is about to reoccur. Except the bad memory keeps replaying, or whatever we are doing to avert a bad memory, is stuck, and replaying. As in compulsive overeating.

EMDR and Peter Levine's more recently introduced Somatic Experiencing therapy work to unlock and release those memories in a way not so easily achieved, let alone accessed, with the rational mind since that is not where the problem has embedded itself.

To understand this more, Levine's "Waking the Tiger"[38], in which he explores and takes his cue from looking at the survival reactions of animals – is worth a read even if you just dip in on the internet.

DEPRESSION / DESPAIR

When feelings become too challenging and we are unable or unwilling to give them their due attention and time in our daily lives, one instinctive way of dealing with them is to bury them out of conscious awareness.

Unfortunately the blocking out or burying tends to have a similar effect across the emotions, generally sapping vitality and potentially manifesting as anything from mild depression, to its more debilitating counterpart, clinical depression.

A particular problem with persistent depression can be a sense of hopelessness and reduced interest in relationships or activities, which

---

[36] EMDR: A therapy developed by Francine Shapiro that works to alleviate symptoms of trauma.

[37] Somatic Experiencing is a form of therapy aimed at relieving and resolving the symptoms of post-traumatic stress disorder (PTSD) and other mental and physical trauma related health problems by focussing on the client's perceived body sensations for somatic experiences.

[38] Waking the Tiger: Healing Trauma – Peter Levine 1997 North Atlantic Books.

along with an accompanying fatigue, might make a person less likely to get help.

Depression can be psychological or biological in origin: sometimes the result of hormonal problems, especially *changing* hormonal levels as, for example, with menopause or post partum depression; or ongoing illness or injury, or a side effect of certain medications. Equally it can be triggered by circumstance or events long in the past. Whichever, overeating at its most mindless perpetuates the anaesthetising or blocking out effect mentioned earlier.

Again, Cognitive Behavioural Therapy is an excellent first port of call for recognising different perspectives, and a shift of mindset. If however this doesn't remotely touch the edge of how you are feeling, once again the therapies mentioned above are well worth investigating.

Benjamin Fry[39], a psychotherapist and author who felt devastated by his depression and, in his own words, stuck in a state of anxiety that had been wrongly diagnosed, describes beautifully his path to wellness at an American clinic which he has now brought to the U.K.

ANXIETY / FEAR

As with the previous example, unconscious overeating may serve to dampen or desensitise the gnawing demand of anxiety and fear, especially when its cause is chronic and quite far back in your personal history. It will be important to check whether the reactions are based on anything real, or emerging with disproportionate regularity in response to events which no longer occur. Anxiety and fear serve as survival mechanisms, but as with post traumatic shock, can be incredibly disruptive if the physical and emotional alarm bells continue to sound at the merest nuance of something which bothers us. By contrast, whilst heightened fear would make it less likely that we'd be eating during an actual emergency, acidity left in the wake of an adrenalin rush is beautifully absorbed by processed carbohydrates.

If the adrenalin secretion is a constant, as with a continual anxiety, however low level, it doesn't take much leap of the imagination to

---

[39] See MailOnline 17th May 2014 and www.khironhouse.com

understand the reaching for comfort foods to literally absorb the acidic overflow...

Yet again Cognitive Behavioural Therapy can work very well with anxieties, enabling a more balanced perspective, though as mentioned above, approaches such as EMDR or Neuro-Linguistic Programming (NLP)[40] and forms of body work can help with the more extreme fears or phobias.

Further, as similarly relevant to the earlier paragraph, while "fight or flight" has worked its way into our everyday language, the bit that is left out as an equally valid survival response is that of playing dead, or freezing. The rabbit in the headlights scenario where unable to think through with the necessary speed, all action is temporarily suspended and we are fixed to the spot. Again, a hallmark of post traumatic shock where a memory is continually replayed, but also perfect ground for a repetitive action to take place, like a stuck record. Areas of highly addictive eating may not necessarily be a reaction to fear, but something none the less, is reacting in the same way, something has become frozen in time.

This kind of eating can be characteristic of a strong addiction to food that is highly resilient and may need professional support. Self condemnation and further shame or anger will never help, and must be gently replaced by compassion, understanding and love. Of course this is always easier said than done. If we were simply able to release unwanted and no longer serving negative emotion, (remembering that our emotions are information, and do serve us, providing they don't get stuck or buried...) we'd all be a whole lot better off, but in the meantime, an understanding of what troubles us goes a long way. It is a lot like sitting close to, and taking the hand of a troubled or upset child: we reassure, we pacify and comfort. We hopefully wouldn't imagine that shouting at, or further shaming the little person, would be of any benefit. But if you're

---

[40] Neuro-linguistic programming (NLP) created by Richard Bandler and John Grinder in the 1970s. Its creators claim a connection between the neurological processes ("neuro"), language ("linguistic") and behavioral patterns learned through experience ("programming") and that these can be changed to achieve specific goals in life.

drying the eyes of that frightened "child" – do not give them chocolate! It's where the story began!

LONGING and (unrequited) LOVE

"What is required for many of us, paradoxical though it may sound, is the courage to tolerate happiness without self sabotage."

Nathaniel Branden[41]

Asked if given only a choice of loving, or being loved, 92% of people I asked chose the former. Testimony to the pursuit of love, indeed just loving, bringing vibrancy and meaning to our lives. Feelings imply for the most part, a connectedness, both with ourselves as well as others. So far so good. The quest for its own sake however, for love or power, or money or status... to fill a gap, becomes problematic. Perhaps given our propensity for thwarting contentment, finding fault with what we do have, or wanting what can't be had or is just beyond reach, it might not be so surprising. Ironically though, the need itself serves the purpose of at least filling that gap, however fleeting. We're back once again to addictions.

A state of need, or *longing* is as all consuming as it is distracting. It can be for power, for security, for a different way of life. The operative word perhaps is **unrequited** which presupposes a longing of whatever kind, and an ongoing anxiety. Longing also implies that we are not fully present in the moment, the here and now. We are in the limbo of an imagined future, which may or may not take place but again creates a gap so easily filled with food.

This longing... can just as easily be happening unconsciously, out of our awareness: an Irish lady I worked with many years ago suddenly realised that almost contrary to expectation, her overeating would automatically self regulate to normal portions whenever she returned home to her mum and family. This was so marked it made her realise that, while otherwise very happy in her relationship with her husband in London, she missed her roots far more than she had accounted for.

---

[41] The Six Pillars of Self Esteem – Nathaniel Branden 1995 Bantam.

Similarly, another lady returning from holiday with her extended family abroad felt an almost unbearable flatness once they had gone and began "graze feeding" throughout the days. Missing people is of course perfectly normal but in bringing the eating reaction and its possible cause into awareness, we are at least more able to take stock and do something about it.

It can be insightful to look at relationships or indeed other significant areas of our lives over the years and notice the weight changes at given times. Where it went up or down and how that corresponded with being alone, or when things went well or badly in some way. Most people will have noticed a marked difference in their eating between for instance, the honeymoon stage of a relationship and its death throes, should that occur… with the contented middle bit often eliciting an increase as old eating habits settle in.

Physiologically, our mouths water as much with physical attraction and desire for intimacy as at the thought of delicious food. It is not hard to see how one can replace the other.

In my later chapter "Lighting your Fire and other distractions", I look at the need to appropriately nourish ourselves on an emotional, and often soulful level, which finds other ways to fill time or need other than eating.

The question is: is any of your eating behaviour to appease a state of need, desire, or an unrequited longing?

-

-

-

-

Does this make a difference if there is a specific focus, or person, or if it is generalized?

-

-

-

WEIGHT AS A BARRIER TO SEX AND INTIMACY – 1
Within a relationship:
In an ongoing, stable relationship weight can easily come from contentment... or raising children or a myriad of other factors. If however, there's a pay off in keeping your partner at bay... you might want to weigh that up against health factors associated with weight gain. Again... not a judgement as to good or bad, simply a matter of becoming aware and taking it on board. Is this what you want? Are you communicating with your partner? Are there other ways of sharing and having intimacy etc etc.... Are you happy enough? Do you want to be in the relationship? Clearly... a potential can of worms here, but on the basis that we ignore things at our peril, that the very drama or fall out or radical action we seek to avoid, is more likely to occur at some stage if we sit on the pressure cooker lid... you might take courage into your hands, lift that lid up just slightly, and have a look at what's going on in your heart. You can't control the other person, or their reactions and response, but taking a good look in your own emotional mirror can be a great place to start!

WEIGHT AS A BARRIER TO SEX AND INTIMACY – 2
Outside a relationship:
Putting on weight or keeping on the weight as a way of insuring we don't attract "trouble" from outside... I've come across more than a few people who have curbed their wild child days in favour of love, family and a stable relationship. Problem can be that if romantic and sexual adventure was a pastime of preference in former days, that yearning for similar excitement can start to reassert itself once more as years go by... and carrying the extra pound... even if we still look good, can make philandering less of an apparent option and a terrific preventative. Plus we get to eat! Similar questions to above... but if you're basically still happy, and especially if there are children in the equation... are there other less dangerous ways to light your fire... other than overeating? Conversely – if carrying the weight isn't affecting health or self esteem and other fall out factors - how you are might work just fine for you!

WEIGHT AS A BARRIER TO SEX AND INTIMACY – 3
Past trauma:

A person who fears sexual experience or intimacy for any reason might unconsciously gain weight to make their body unattractive. It's an instinctive self protecting mechanism rather than by design. If you have had a painful or traumatic sexual experience on a physical or emotional level, your unconscious may be saying "no more of this" and making yourself as unappealing as possible. Ask yourself "How safe do I feel sexually when I am at or nearing my perfect weight?" I've noticed on occasion with clients that if someone has been sexually assaulted or abused, in their past, there can be real problems returning anywhere near the weight at the time of the event. It is rarely conscious but rather, psychosomatic, i.e. that link between body and mind which sends off alarms signals at the onset of danger[42]. If this is linked with a previous weight, you may find yourself forever returning, instinctively, to a "safer" weight, i.e. one that is not the same, doesn't act as a "marker", and maybe less perceivably attractive. If you suspect this is the case, you might consider getting gentle help in alleviating the "stuck" fear and memory which is creating a fight or flight reaction. Or more pertinently, the frozen in the headlights reaction. Be mindful however, that it goes at a pace you feel comfortable with. These days you do *not* have to go through the trauma of resurrecting or re-living the experience more than you already do. There is fantastic work out there now with Post Traumatic Stress (PTSD)[43] and Somatic Experiencing (SE). Trauma specialist Babette Rothschild[42] is a leader in the field while residential workshops such as Growth and Transition[44] created by the late Elisabeth Kubler-Ross enable a safe, contained and supportive environment to work through whatever has kept you stuck. Of course you may want to consider whether things are in fact best left alone, or whether an issue from the past is still festering and causing problems. If you're still affected by something, reacting to it, then it isn't really in the past: it's still here, now. It's cast its shadow into

---

[42] The Body Remembers by Babette Rothschild – W W Norton & Co. Nov 2000.
[43] www.somatictraumatherapy.com
[44] www.growthandtransition.com

189

your future and is banging on the door in the present. I am not an advocate for needlessly digging up the past – but I do operate on a Need to Function Well Enough basis. So if your mental, emotional and / or physical health is suffering and your wellbeing is compromised, you might want to sort it – at least enough to get your life back.

WEIGHT AS A SOCIAL BARRIER

For many people, putting on weight can detract from full enjoyment as they feel self conscious and more preoccupied with how they look and how they might be judged.

For some however, the extra weight actually acts as a layer of protection: if you fear meeting new people and participating in social situations, might you be using those extra pounds as a barrier to keep people from getting to know you? Ironically, when the self esteem is low, many people feel both invisible within the layers of fat and over conspicuous at the same time. Working with self acceptance and beginning to value who and how you are, will be key to making headway here.

* * *

Eating behaviours may emerge automatically to plug any emotional hole, so whether the cause is toxic and has its roots entrenched in childhood family history, or whether a chronic backlog of unacknowledged anger or grief, this will need at least to be taken on board for any weight loss to be of value at a later stage. Otherwise the automatic eating will simply re-emerge to do the emotional hole-plugging job it performs very well. But always at a cost.

Ask yourself:

What feeling is strongest when I reach for food which I do not actually need? Remember how you feel after you've eaten might be different to how you felt beforehand: you may for example, feel guilty or angry or upset with yourself an hour or so after you ate, but that probably wasn't the emotion that initially set you off.

190

-

-

What thoughts are uppermost in my mind?

-

-

Where is the feeling in my body? Am I responding physically in any way? I.e. is my breathing shallow? Does my head or back ache, etc?

-

-

Do I know the source of how I am feeling?

-

-

Can you think of situations or events that led to how you are feeling?

-

-

Even if you are unsure, start to collect that evidence of the link between situations, events, thoughts, feelings, and your overeating.

If you believe you are not good at self reflection, the clue will always be in the overeating behaviour! It's like a treasure hunt in reverse, so work backward from there!

When you find yourself eating without being hungry, **ask yourself:**

… and this helps me – how?

Or:

Will this change anything? Will this change how I feel, or the situation?

And again:

Will I be pleased with my choice in two hours time?

Remember at all times, this is not about good or bad or right or wrong, you are simply collecting information. Over time this will help you make better choices, ahead of the fact rather than after.

All hindsight becomes foresight over time.

The Physically Driven Spectrum

THE PHYSICAL SPECTRUM

WELLBEING / GENERAL HEALTH

←——————————————————————→

Very healthy   *Health issues*

Well   *Illness*

Pain free   *Need for pain management*

Good equilibrium   *Out of balance*

Good activity levels   *Low activity levels*

Full mobility   *Impaired mobility*

Low stress levels   *High stress levels*

Hormonal cycles / time of the month

Regular   *Irregular*

Hormonal cycles / time of life, menopause

Young   *Middle aged*   *Elderly*

Refreshed   *Frequently tired*

Good sleep patterns   *Bad sleep patterns*

WEIGHT

←——————————————————————→

Excellent weight   *Erratic weight management*
management

194

Eating Behaviours and the Physically driven spectrum.

Just as our energy levels, and how we are physically, are impacted reciprocally by the circumstances of our lifestyle and emotional wellbeing, so too does the optimal functioning of our bodies affect in turn, our outlook and who we are. Our biography in short, becomes our biology, and so the repercussions continue.

As you detail in the information from each of the spectrums which will make up your personal eating behaviour blueprint, the knock on effects between each should become increasingly apparent.

Looking at the chart above, where would you say you fit? If any of them vary, for how long, when, and do you know why the change? Do you tend more often toward good sleep, good health etc, or the not so good? When we look in the next chapter at the collective mix of all three spectrums, everything comes into consideration. As I continue to reiterate, often the smallest change can shift the whole dynamic for the better.

Our start point however, is that we do need to eat.

Real hunger v emotional hunger...

A main challenge here is that emotional hunger easily masks itself as real physical hunger. The difference may not be obvious until you have managed your eating behaviours for a while and have a gauge of what for you is more normal. One of my group, Jane, had been almost exemplary in keeping to revised eating plans till the day she had a row with her partner. She disclosed her horror at finding herself "gorging from the fridge" before she "came to" and realised what she was doing. On reflection, this had been a regular and pretty well automatic reaction from her in her past, but the extent to which it was borne of emotion rather than hunger was only now startlingly clear and something of a revelation. Reason enough to check with care what fits with the emotional spectrum.

Ask yourself:
Am I really hungry?

Tiredness... fatigue...

Although I have not collated statistical evidence – my years of experience have made me certain that levels of tiredness, and that includes emotional fatigue, has to be a key ingredient in undermining any diet, or stable weight maintenance.

There are already motorway signs everywhere attesting "Tiredness kills!" to the point that it is a criminal offence if nodding off contributes to an accident. And while there are no legal implications, perhaps neon signs around cafes flashing "Tiredness tips the scales!!" might be a great reminder! (I shouldn't think food outlets would be up for this novel drive but perhaps one for local councils – with a knack for the self righteous, perish the thought!)

Most of us if up early, have a mid afternoon energy dip as glucose levels drop slightly, but being tired is akin to an *all* day dip, and over and above the body's desire to eat something, resolve to hold back from anything less than biscuits, cake, bread and crisps is likely to be at an all time low. (A moot point to mention that fruit and plenty of water really does help...)

Focus is the frontrunner...

When someone reneges on their eating plan, I don't so much ask why they ate, as how come they lost focus. Planning is pivotal, but to maintain the planning, we need focus. Focus is lost through lack of sleep, and prolonged lack of sleep all the more so. Whether or not something can be done to enable more or better sleep will of course vary individually, but if you are someone permanently affected by some level of tiredness... look to redress this as much as you can *before* you even think of dieting. You may well find that the renewed resolve to hold back from titbits alone, has a marked effect on your eating behaviour and subsequent weight loss.

Double whammy...

As lack of sleep affects equally our stress levels and emotional wellbeing, you are likely to feel the odds overwhelmingly stacked against you if you are an emotional eater, even when bright and bushy tailed. Sorting the sleep issue may then not be an option and it may even be worth considering a change of job… I guess it depends on how badly your health is coming into question if the weight is soaring…?

My own experience working as long haul cabin crew for years was a perpetual battle with a voracious appetite, as I rarely made up for working through time zones as well as through nights. Exacerbated by my work environment (social spectrum) with its on tap provision of edibles at hotels or in the galley, and kid yourself not, the food from B.A. first class is well, pretty good, it was hardly surprising that the weight fell off once I stopped flying.

Never underestimate the power of feeling fully refreshed! (Or changing your job!)

Ask yourself:

- Am I tired a lot of the time?

- All of the time?

- Some of the time?

- When – as a rule… i.e. later in the week? Sunday mornings?

- Is it accumulative from work, stress etc, or from late nights?

- How much sleep do you feel best on as a rule?

- What is the minimum you need to feel good enough?

- Is the quality of your sleep better when you go to bed earlier?

- Can you *get* to bed earlier?

- Is the quality of your sleep better when you eat earlier?

- Can you eat earlier?

- If you eat late to share dinner with your partner, can you make this a lighter meal?

- Is the quality of your sleep better when you don't drink alcohol?

- Can you limit your alcohol intake at least some days of the week?

Tip: As most of us are not good at having "just one", it's a lot easier not drinking at all certain days of the week, say Monday to Thursday. It quickly becomes an established routine and a good habit.

Tip: Offering to drive means you stay alcohol free and are thanked for it as well!

What small changes are you *willing* to make?
What small changes are you *able* to make?

Whatever you do, notice and *write down* any improvements, both in how you feel, but more measurably with regard to your eating habits. Do not imagine you will remember, we are mostly far too busy and besides tend to have selective memories! Remember you are doing invaluable detective work, so you need to *collect the evidence*! It's like doing the accounts and this alone will provide you with the leverage to continue making the effort!

Hormonal cycles and times of the month...
Even if you are not a great comfort eater, the hormonal cycle affects many women emotionally and in addition, the body's apparent need for anything sweet just prior to, and alongside the onset of menstruation, can be overwhelming.

Ask yourself:
- Do you have a chocolate or sugar fest of some kind, then end up carrying on so it carries over into the week or the rest of the month?
- Could you substitute the sweet stuff with healthier "fixes"?
  (See "Tricks of the Trade: Food wisdom and curbing the urge" later on).
- Could you put something in place that enables you to go back to normal eating sooner rather than later? For example instead of thinking you've "blown it", actually allowing yourself the downtime once a month on the basis you revert...? It's then guilt free *and* sustainable.

198

Polycystic Ovarian syndrome...

Worse, if you suffer from PCOS, the cycle can be far longer than the usual 5 to 7 days, prolonging the whole effect and creating an emotional rollercoaster that can make life hell for anyone who already uses food to cope.

The latter will need specialist advice from a GP but ensuring your staple intake is nutritionally balanced and complete should be prioritized. Many of the omega 3/6/9 range of vitamins, along with primrose and starflower oils really can make a noticeable difference for some women.

Tip: If your likelihood of maintaining any sensible eating during your cycle is low to zero, and the increasing weight is simply compounding your distress, what can work well is taking the weight increase every month into account, then working out a more moderate, or restricted eating plan during the rest of the month which restores the balance. It's a version of *paying it forward* (see Tricks of the Trade) and along with doing the job, restores sanity to your life and a sense of being back in charge. Again, you'll need to collect the evidence and do the maths!

Additionally, although hormonal problems can induce a gain in weight, weight gain in itself can create hormonal imbalance, and many people find an easing of symptoms and hormonal rebalancing as their overeating is modified and a healthier weight resumed.

Testimony to this has to be the number of women who have taken on board quite a radical, though nutritionally complete, very low calorie diet, (VLCD) in order to lose weight to begin IVF and have then become pregnant before treatment even began. Three of my own clients, each of whom had been unable to conceive for up to six years and were advised to lose at least 3 stone, became pregnant within three to six months of joining a group – and each had a baby. Information regarding this within the weight loss and weight management company for whom I worked for many years was, if not actually statistically significant, enough that many of us would advise clients not wishing to increase their progeny to take precautions and not assume they'd be safe!

Hormonal cycles, lifestyle and work schedules...

On the basis that the monthly cycle compounded by a mood change, further exacerbates eating patterns, it can be worthwhile to avoid coupling this, where at all possible, with even more stress. You may not have an iota of choice but if, for example, you have an important event and there is choice as to the exact date, avoid the overlap, if you can. Attempting to maintain a diet of any kind is already susceptible to "I've blown it", but a combination of that important interview, a problematic relative coming to stay, and time of the month is probably going to take stress levels to combustion point. And bang goes another diet. Just a thought.

Hormonal cycles and the menopause...

Should you have a considerable amount of weight to lose there are two major reasons for treating yourself to a seriously new eating regime *before* the menopause is fully under way if you are at all able:

The first is that as oestrogen levels drop, so too does the elasticity of the skin. Although skin type as well as bone structure makes a difference, and I have seen a person in their seventies look better, in my opinion, than a much younger person with a different frame, it still bodes better if done earlier. Further, dramatic weight loss can induce the same kind of hair shedding as pregnancy, or for that matter during the colder weather, when the body is trying to conserve its energy, and although hair grows back, I have noticed a stronger effect when age and stress levels combine with hormonal change. This is however, only my personal observation, and I would reiterate it is the *change* in hormones which seems to be key.

The second is that the menopause is a *transition,* which for many hastens the end of a major part of their lives with far reaching implications. It can herald as much as anything a change in how we see ourselves, and if we use food as a coping mechanism, this might prove a challenging time to let go of that too in trying to lose weight. It could feel like one bereavement too many.

All of this said and done, the guide must always be whatever you feel is right at the time. You are absolutely your best guide, and context is everything!

Although dieting can affect the period cycle, sometimes disappearing for the duration and at other times reappearing after a long absence, there have been no adverse effects from long term dieting **providing** your diet is nutritionally balanced and you are not, in effect, starving yourself. This is very different to the catastrophic reduction of intake symptomatic of anyone with history of anorexia which can adversely affect the hormonal cycle.

Illness / Injury / Physical Disability / Impaired Mobility…
I've wrapped all these under one heading because the two main problems that arise are the same:

The first is that due to restricted activity levels, and simply not being able to move around as much or as quickly, far less is burnt off and weight gain can happen with minimal intake. Which means that what you eat and how much you eat is, just to add to your woes, far more critical than someone with full mobility.

The second is that even people who do not especially have issues with food can end up comfort eating under the circumstances. Physical as well as emotional distress can really up the ante and the temptation to indulge has a powerful pull, even if only to fill time less easily spent otherwise. Having to eat "sensibly" can feel almost impossible to keep to and a contradiction in terms. However much you may feel eating is the only enjoyment you are getting, you may want to check it doesn't create an additional burden to your health, or lengthen your recovery process.

The extent to which you are physically immobilized or in pain, and the circumstances surrounding it, including any current medication will of course not only affect what you can and can't do, but your mindset and emotional wellbeing as well.

If whatever limits your mobility is not something which is likely to improve, it will be far more necessary to take things into hand sooner rather than later. Again, easier said than done, but if quality of life depends on it, the inner reserves people draw upon can be as extraordinary as they are moving and inspiring. What will be necessary is some creative decision making, and for that to be possible you will need an overview of the big picture, i.e. what your options are and what's at risk. It doesn't always mean we are able to rise above ourselves and act in our own best interests, but at least having some idea of the odds will allow us to prioritize one way or the other.

Opting over and again for the treat at the end of each day may be no different to the 90% of the nation who regain weight, but you may have far more immediately at stake. As I make plain in the chapter on "Goal Setting and Setting your Intention", there's nothing like a wake up call...

The lifesaver for someone whose reduced mobility is temporary, is that you do at least have a time frame, and knowing that you can offload any weight gained once you're back to normal provides some light at the end of the tunnel. The downside of that glimmer of hope though, can be less to stop you doing real damage in the meantime.

Tip: In order to not give up hope entirely and moreover for your eating behaviours to hold steady, especially with such a tight rein, it works well to have *some* gratification to look forward to.

As *I* have problems with ***portion control*** I have two ways of maintaining a steady weight, which works for me and has worked for many of my clients:

First: 4 to 5 days a week I keep to that wonderful euphemism, sensible eating. But in order to keep my monkey mind from going on the prowl, I have to know something good is ahead.

Eating something small, however mind-blowingly delicious, is over and done with far too soon. Any self respecting gastronome, or, someone trapped by circumstance, needs just a wee bit longer than the eating equivalent of wham bam and thank you ma'am. This is *not* just about physical satiation. It's about emotional fullness. So, once a day, only, I will eat for at least 25 minutes. It has to have a crunch, and it always has a really good "hit."

The "crunch" may be a crisper type of salad, and I mean a bowlful, or it may be croutons, but it does the trick, as does the "hit" which could be a lacing of parmesan or a few olives or an omelette or a good sized portion of sea bass ... whatever... It is however, and this is important, still in the "sensible" eating category. But not dying of boredom means you're more likely to hold that balance and keep to your plan.

Second: banging the gratification drum once again... and providing you are not on a weight *loss* regime, knowing you can have a pretty good time for a couple of days once a week gives you strength to hold on. Somehow there is hope in the distance, on a weekly basis, and that means you are *less* likely to throw in the eating behaviour towel and hell to the consequence.

Sedentary lifestyle, work etc.

You may or may not have choice in this, but if you have choice, *use it.*

Whilst no amount of exercise will actually offset eating - past a certain point, the reverse is that something about keeping even a little bit active, not only burns off some of the calories but far more importantly, tends to create what I call the *virtuous mindset.* And if you're in that virtuous mindset, you're a little bit less likely to be filling time with titbits.

Where there is no apparent choice however, you might want to decide how much any surplus weight, (especially the centrally deposited fat which is more likely with continued sitting...) is jeopardising your health and quality of life, and see where change can be made.

Ask yourself:

- Is eating surplus to my body's needs going to make things a lot worse if my weight keeps increasing?

- If my reduced mobility is temporary, how likely *am* I to remedy things once back to normal? (In other words has your eating always contributed to weight issues, or have you always been fairly slim? That'll be your clue.)

- On the basis that going up from zero is something, can I introduce even five or ten minutes a day more activity than I am doing at the moment?

Tip: In the "*anything up from zero is good*" book of philosophy... anything...even *five minutes* of *any* kind of movement which is up from your usual, will be a move for the better. Better still, make it while watching TV or listening to the radio every day and a routine starts to get set.

Tip: If you are unaccustomed to much activity, do not attempt a vigorous bout of heroics. *Use the floor* or a chair with a good back, as your support.

Tip: Making changes like using the stairs instead of a lift, or parking your car or getting off the train a couple of stops earlier and walking the rest of the way to work, is again Up from Zero and starts the ball rolling. Anything to keep fitter than you are right now, even if it's twirling your feet or running on the spot for a minute, is a step in the right direction. If you're very out of practise even the smallest amount of movement is going to make a difference. Go with what feels right to you and in keeping with your energy. Nothing else counts.

Tip: Do something you love. If you hate the gym, don't join. What's the point. If you find the thought of something sucks the life blood through your eyeballs when you're full of good intent, what will happen once the motivation slips.

Make a list, now, of anything you love which includes any kind of movement. A walk in the park. Salsa. Zumba. Swimming. Yoga. Pilates. Tennis. Kicking the ball around. Cycling. And the rest...

When less is more - lack of time:
N.E.A.T. and up from zero...
Apropos the above, there was a wonderful Horizon programme with Michael Moseley[45] in 2012 in which he tested out the difference even short bursts of exercise made to the entire physical system. The results were

---

[45] Horizon 2011/2012 "The Truth about Exercise." (also Horizon 2012/ 2013 "Eat, Fast, Live Longer").

fairly remarkable and totally positive. The beauty of N.E.A.T which stands for Non Exercising Activity Thermogenesis, is that **anything** and everything counts. So if you are one of the workbound or housebound, finding even *ten minutes a day* really does make a difference, and again, is one up from zero![46]

Ask yourself:

- Is there **any** new movement you can introduce in your current circumstances?
- Could you start with just five minutes a day?
- Could you up to ten minutes a day after a week?
- Could you up to 15 minutes a day, after a fortnight?

When less is more - impaired mobility:

When I first taught yoga in my local area, I was concerned as to my level of fitness and keeping up with adepts. I need not have worried. Out from under the woodwork came the elderly, in their droves, like some kind of reverse Pied Piper effect, and all of a sudden my daytime class was half full of seventy to ninety year olds. Initially a little downhearted at the necessarily revised shift in pace and level, I was astonished as much by the power of minimized movement with careful use of chair or floor, as the power of focus on breathing. I am not suggesting miracles here, but the visible improvement within weeks was a lesson to me. I am passing this now onto you! It doesn't have to be yoga: any small movement, or position, that goes with the flow of your body, generally breathing *out* with exertion, and *in* as you "let go", can vitalize areas of stuck energy in your body *as well as* helping to still the mind. But remember, no heroics!

At the end of the Goal Setting chapter I included "Letter to my Body" which includes all that your body has done for you, despite our protestations, and how we might value it better. If you didn't do so before,

---

[46] FastExercise: the simple secret of high intensity training by Michael Mosley with Peta Bee. First Atria Books 2014.

and any of the Physical Spectrum is particularly relevant, you might want to take another look and consider how you *might* better serve your body, so that *it* serves *you* best!

What do you want?
What are you *willing* to do?
What are you *able* to do?

Putting It All Together
and Identifying
High Risk Combinations

PUTTING IT ALL TOGETHER
and IDENTIFYING HIGH RISK COMBINATIONS

By now you will recognize how the need for *structure,* together with our quest for *meaning,* combined with the desire for *stimulus* and *emotional comfort,* on *top* of how we're feeling *physically* at any given time, packs a more than potent punch: stirred together, we habituate with insidious ease into automatic reaction and levels of addiction. It's like a kind of Holy Grail, held in place in a chalice of lifestyle, culture and environment, and bound with the nectar of habit...

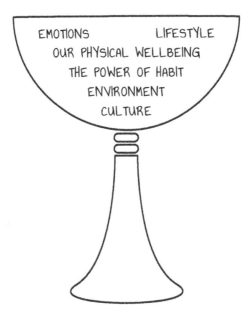

EMOTIONS   LIFESTYLE
OUR PHYSICAL WELLBEING
THE POWER OF HABIT
ENVIRONMENT
CULTURE

"A GREAT BIG CHALICE HOLDING IT ALL TOGETHER."

Which bit of the combined matrix of lifestyle and circumstance, emotions, physical wellbeing and food itself will be the easiest bit to change first?

It's easy to see how if we've become stuck into repetitive eating patterns, it isn't just a matter of counting the calories. Good or bad, it takes little to begin a habit which given everything else going on, becomes quickly entrenched. It starts out as a newly trod path and over time becomes the equivalent of a well used motorway: when eventually we try to stop, the path of least resistance, the fall down the same old hole is like going back along that same motorway, which has far greater pull, far more usage. As we saw earlier, that is how a habit is *meant* to be.

It is *meant* to operate at the unconscious level. Which is at once its beauty and our nemesis! In order to stop doing the same old same old with the blink of an eye in a New York minute, we have to become increasingly alert to ourselves.

Doing the detective is about noticing the steps that combine more often than not to precipitate an eating reaction that might otherwise make little sense.

Sometimes the tipping point is so mundane it is overlooked. Other times it may be several days prior to the eating behaviour becoming erratic, so again it is missed.

One client some years back had held her weight well for months till she began once again overeating, without apparent reason. Initially she said there had been no change in her circumstances during the previous seven days. What transpired however, was that her beloved dog of many years had died three weeks before, followed by an argument with her mother which had badly upset her. As she spoke, her more than understandable upset was apparent and she realised she'd been desperate for days to eat for comfort as she used to. It was like a pressure cooker of emotion building up and searching for an outlet.

Another lady was doing equally well till her small grandson became seriously ill the same week as a particularly gruelling dental appointment. Traumatised by the ordeal of an over vigorous root extraction she lacked her usual resilience, and concern for her son's child hit what seemed like an especially raw spot. Yet until I drew the combining events up on a flip chart, she couldn't see why she'd been so "weak willed."

The combination might be simply a case of being too tired, being over bored in a job you feel you can't change, or a longer period at home with temptation all around. Whatever the situation, you need to add all the relevant aspects of the social, emotional and physical spectrums that relate to you at the time. You will recognise the main triggers and tripwires quickly enough.

You might find a way of putting to paper your "combined events" that works better for you, but for the moment have a look at the illustrations overleaf: What you're looking for are the situations or emotions that take your eating behaviours to a critical tipping point. A straw that breaks the camel's back. People often minimize what is upsetting them because it can sound as though we are without backbone or can't cope. But the issue is simply one of looking as dispassionately and objectively as possible at *what is going on.* When we assign judgement we are likely to miss the point and the valuable information it brings. The more accurately we can pinpoint whatever got the ball rolling, the more likely we are to be able to make a change that works even minimally. At the very least, a more objective recognition can help lessen the self recrimination which usually makes us reach even more for food as comfort.

Thinking back, ask yourself: What does food do for you? How does it help you? When and why do you most "overuse" it? To pass time?

To concentrate, chew the cud, reflect....? To procrastinate and put things off? To celebrate? To create the illusion of space between things to do....? To provide the illusion of emotional comfort..?

Then as you start to think about combinations which for you create ongoing risk, have a look at the questions below:

Why do I eat at these times?
What purpose is the food serving?
If your actions / body could speak, what would the dialogue be?
How would the conversation go?
What does your eating mask, or cover up?
What alternatives might there be?
If you were watching your best friend do this, how would you see the situation?
Will you be pleased with your choice in two hours time?

Is the emotional solace this food provides going to change anything?
Do you want whatever it provides in the immediate moment....more ...
than what being slimmer and healthier will provide?

It can be useful to draw a mind map or circle diagrams on a weekly basis or *whenever you cannot quite reconcile the strength of an eating habit* with what is going on. Lightbulb moments happen regularly when circumstances are drawn up and made easily visible. Over time you will become increasingly familiar with the factors which, added together, create a High Risk tipping point. Include whatever is going on today, this week, this month, and what might be more of a general backdrop. Someone who has a demanding day to day existence, (most parents for example?!) can often omit this simply because it seems the norm, yet what has been overlooked is an already present level of ongoing stress, or depletion of energy. It isn't about excuse making here. It's about looking at facts and seeing all the bits that make up an equation. This is the heart of your detective work where following the crumbs as it were, leads to far greater insight and possibly realising that even something small can make a change for the better.

As the emotional, circumstantial and physical factors start to add up and overlap, our reserves can begin to diminish until our resilience hits an all time low - and we "fill up" in response to this.

It really is worth noticing and recording, over time, what combinations set off an attack that is recoverable, from which you can indeed pull yourself sooner rather than later back from the brink, which combinations have a more prolonged effect, and those which set off overeating patterns which become rollercoasters and create longer term damage. Becoming increasingly aware of this means you can start to work ahead of the fact.

Remember though, this is not about having to work to change the seemingly impossible: it's about making whatever changes are feasible so you don't keep hitting the critical tipping point. It's keeping that pressure at a manageable level, and yes, if there is a chronically underlying issue that you realise would do well to be altered, you can take time to make that choice from a more informed perspective.

Bear in mind too, that what you assume might be the main reasons may change subtly over time to reveal something surprisingly different. The obvious is never obvious enough.

Ask yourself:
What is the *smallest* change I can make which will have the *greatest* effect?

Moderate effort - maximum impact!

PUTTING IT ALL TOGETHER
IDENTIFYING HIGH RISK COMBINATIONS

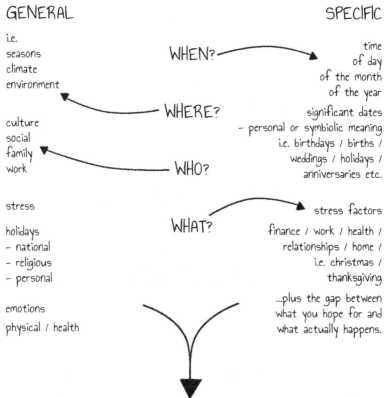

GENERAL   SPECIFIC

i.e.
seasons   WHEN?   time
climate   of day
environment   of the month
                                                       of the year

culture   WHERE?   significant dates
social   - personal or symbiolic meaning
family   i.e. birthdays / births /
work   WHO?   weddings / holidays /
                                                    anniversaries etc.

stress   stress factors
                                               finance / work / health /
holidays   WHAT?   relationships / home /
- national   i.e. christmas /
- religious   thanksgiving
- personal

emotions   ...plus the gap between
physical / health   what you hope for and
                                                what actually happens.

Where the habit hits the hardest.
i.e. time, place associations =
the conditional response...

DESIRE + REWARD + REPETITION = HABIT

IDENTIFYING HIGH RISK COMBINATIONS

An overabundance of overlapping areas means you have a high risk combination. Energy wise you are on a "low reserve" and about to "run on empty". This creates a CRITICAL TIPPING POINT when almost anything can become the last straw. There is usually a time factor here, a few hours at least, if we are alert, before a Big Time Blowout at which point it's as though you're in your own blind spot: no longer *you* doing the eating.

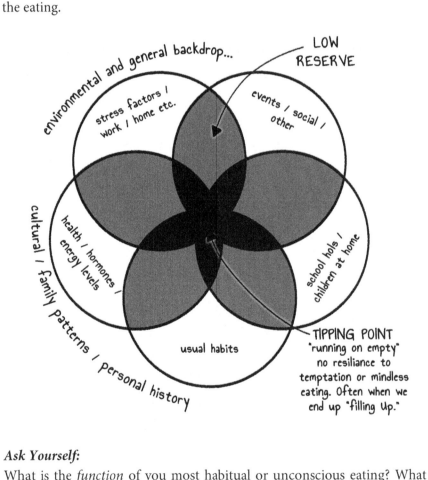

Ask Yourself:

What is the *function* of you most habitual or unconscious eating? What does it *serve*? Your words and language will provide strong clues re: WHAT? WHEN? WHO? WHY?

THE MAGIC MATRIX

So far we have been exploring what adds up to create a High Risk combination. The Magic Matrix on the other hand is whatever might represent the near ideal situation for you to maintain healthy eating patterns, a good relationship with food, and hence a stable weight at the right end of the scales.

Four of the main factors here are the times at which you eat, the time at which you go to bed and whether you get enough sleep, the amount of activity you are able to include in any day or week, and your optimal food choices.

Many years ago during my travels I spent four weeks at an Indian hill station. I rose daily around 8am and after an hour's yoga would have coconut water and papaya for breakfast, dhal and fish for lunch around 1pm, and dinner around 6pm. The freshness of the food, my choice of timing, the level of activity and ok, the absence of stress felt like the magical combination for a far healthier way of eating. It was nigh on perfect!

Later – over the years I ran a business from home, one of the luxuries was "managing" my eating and again the timing. While Saturdays entailed back to back groups throughout the day, I always had 45 minutes for soup and salad or suchlike around 1.30 pm. Other than the rare emergency nobody came in during this time. I learnt early that, however tempting it might be to use the additional time to fit in more work – it was a non-negotiable: without it I would get horribly over tired and over hungry and end up on a choc and carb fest the minute people had left late afternoon. The introduction of the light lunch carried me through, enabling a more measured approach to the evening meal (as well as insuring professional authenticity!).

Finding the right combination *may* presuppose sufficient calm and reduced stress levels but it can work *both* ways. Becoming able to return to a combination that works for you may in turn facilitate an improved wellbeing and all that stems from it.

Ask yourself:

Given total choice of what would most likely create a best imagined relationship with food, and help stabilise your weight:

What would be your choice of meal times?

What time would you go to bed at night / how much sleep would you have?

What kind of activity would you most enjoy that would keep your body healthy enough and burn off at least a base level of calorific energy!

What would be your choice of food?

You might want to differentiate between the week and weekends.

Have a look at the Matrix Triangle on the next page.

The Magic Matrix

Whatever combinations prove to be as near ideal as you can get to maintain a healthy relationship with food and a healthy sufficiently stable weight.

The 'ingredients' may vary but are likely to include:

Meal *Timing*, Optimal Food Choices, Enough Activity and Enough Sleep.

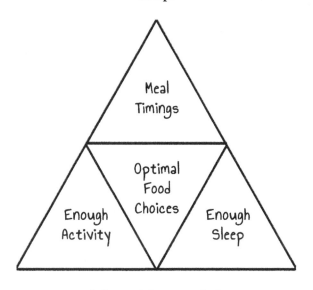

What might yours be?

You may have little to no reference for what would comprise your ideal combination, but think back to any time when your eating moderated even briefly. If this is seriously off your radar, then keep alert from now on for any time, however short lived, in which something about your day or your week feels balanced, in a relative state of harmony, and is reflected in your eating behaviour. Or when conversely, your eating behaviour elicits a greater wellbeing because you feel happier about your success.

When this happens, and it will, make sure you keep a record of everything that made up your day or your week. Rather like my sojourn at Ooty in Southern India, you may find it is a period of rest or holiday that elicits the longed for moderation but it still counts as a template.

That template can be looked at and implemented even in part into some of your daily living. It's a bit like *copy and paste* on your computer. However you choose to see it, it's setting a precedent for a better way of living and being.

You may already know what makes up your *magical matrix* or it may be a work in progress. Whichever, keep something within view that reminds you daily of what you're aspiring towards.

It is also useful to do a High Risk combination drawing on a weekly basis and compare one with the other.

As we go through the next chapters you'll find more ways to recognize when you're reverting to type with eating habits, and other ways to help you get through when you do.

PART 3:
STRATEGIES FOR COPING

Prioritizing in action:
DO, DELEGATE or DUMP!

The basis for Cognitive Behavioural Therapy is that where there is a negative knock on effect between situations and how we experience life, i.e. our thoughts, feelings and behaviours, an intervention which helps us to think differently and have a better perspective can really turn things around. After all, context is everything, and it is true that it's not what you see – but how you see it.

A great if over simplified example of this might be where one of the mums in my group was forever depressed about her ability to cope, and berating her lack of organisation. To put you in the picture, she had four children between 6 and 12, one of them had special needs, and she worked full time. You can see where we're going here.

What was manifestly apparent as we unpicked what for her might be an average day, was that considering her schedule and the amount she had to do, with a day that began around 5.30 am and was cram packed till ten or eleven pm ish ... anyone in her position would have been hard put to do much better.

As each of us hearing her situation came to a similar conclusion, (a bonus of being nine or more in a group, is that it's difficult to negate or dismiss as one person's point of view...) her relief was visible: ok, the amount she had to do hadn't changed, but her perception of her being inadequate as a person and a mother had really been eating into her, and the two or three glasses of wine a night plus several bags of crisps to "take the edge off things"... during the only time she would finally sit and relax before midnight...had been piling on the pounds for months. Several of the group were also working mums which helped the validation.

Bringing to mind yet again our swinging metal spheres, no matter what you do, everything affects everything else and there is a knock on effect impacting every part of your life. Every choice, and that includes the choice of how you react or respond, makes a difference. It's infinitesimal and works to the nth degree without exception. The upside is a kind of worldwide web of interconnectedness with all beings great and small, a butterfly effect that whatever the circumstances gives us some small charge of which way destinies might tip; the downside, if you see it as such, is having to come away from blame and being mindfully accountable for all we do.

On the global stage, Nelson Mandela remains one of the most currently well known examples of this in action, admired and revered not merely for his work in finally tipping anti apartheid scales but even more because, without his extraordinary ability to forgive and put his anger by for the better good, the whole story would have been so tragically different.

Returning to the commonplace however... the process of this knock on effect can be drawn as a line, but actually it's a circle with a loop that can become worse and worse or better and better. Or sometimes it might just go round and round until something gets thrown in to improve or worsen. That something can often be overwhelming fatigue and a quality of sleep, increasingly impaired by alcohol, as with our mum.

It's that **chain reaction** in motion again. In linear form it would have situations and what is going on for you at one end, with behaviour at the other. Because what we are concerned with is the end effect on our eating behaviours, I put **eating behaviours** at the end of the line.

Situations / how you see it / your thoughts / how you feel / what you end up doing

Drawn as a circle you can see more easily how what you end up doing, i.e. over eating, in turn affects the next situation:

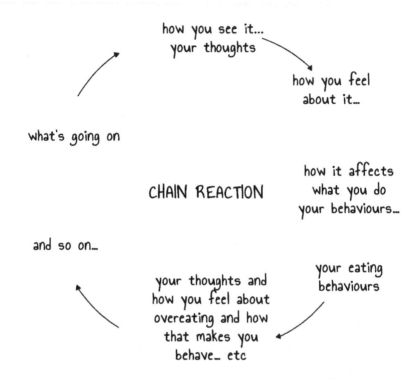

how you see it...
your thoughts

how you feel
about it...

what's going on

CHAIN REACTION

how it affects
what you do
your behaviours...

and so on...

your eating
behaviours

your thoughts and
how you feel about
overeating and how
that makes you
behave... etc

Coming back to our mum – she was having a light bulb moment with regard to her not being such a dreadful person after all... but that didn't change her being tired and overloaded. Seeing something from a fresh perspective is immensely freeing... and may at times – if we consider many of the amputees returning from war zones – be our only recourse to healing and becoming whole again within ourselves... but so too is a genuine change in a situation.

Rosy (our mum) was feeling a bit better about herself with the support of the group... but if the tiredness and with it the eating and weight issues, continued, it would be all too normal to end up feeling down about herself again. I asked whether any of her workload could be lessened and whether any of her day could be done differently: as Rosy spoke, what came across in equal measure was how tight a control she believed she needed to have with the housework and the home, and how much of the day she spent putting off her most hated tasks and how that really took it out of her.

Also, that she really did have too much to accomplish each and every day.

Three questions emerged: what could she best do first in her day, to not spend so much time putting off the inevitable, what might she let someone else do, and what could she in fact let go of.

What could be **prioritized,** what could be **delegated,** what could be **dumped.**

Lest you are wondering how this relates to eating behaviours, though hopefully you are with me on this, the answer is inextricably: whilst obesity numbers are rising so alarmingly that a normalising of emotional eating has to be taken on board, a vast number of people whose weight might not otherwise be an issue have lifestyles with very little room for regular healthy eating. Stress levels and fatigue compound, and the cycle worsens by the day. A perfectly working chain reaction.

Many situations seem unchangeable. The stuff of life. Much of what you will have put down on your own Social Spectrum, and many of the feelings that are particularly challenging from the Emotional Spectrum. Add physical and health issues and we really set tinder to the fire. But few situations are 100 per cent *un*changeable. There is almost always some tiny thing which can be brought forward, delegated, or left out entirely and all we need for those eating behaviours to moderate, even minimally, is to find a tipping point. It is possible that if you fall more heavily to the emotional eating end of the equation, they may not be so easily moderated by a mere practical manoeuvre, but on the basis of a reciprocal loop between circumstances, who, where, what and when, and emotional sensitivity, there will still be *an* effect. And it all adds up.

What transpired with Rosy, as with many of us, was a reluctance to delegate some of the household chores on the basis of needing a job well done, and a concern about letting go of ironing her husband's shirts despite his saying he'd be perfectly happy to do them, because it was part of her "wifey thing".

Bear in mind her full time job which doesn't leave her an exorbitant amount of time once she's home every day.

I've chosen this example because, without being psychological rocket science, other agendas complicate the issue of "just delegating or letting go.." yet typify the **kind** of entanglements which once realised, can be easily worked with.

What we looked at, along with others in the group who brought in their own examples, was the worst possible outcome of Rosy letting her husband do the dishwasher every evening, and her very keen to be grown up twelve year old sorting out her own clothes for school each day and making her own bed.

What transpired was a level of guilt for not being a sufficiently at home mum and almost invariably arriving later than her husband at nights, after work, hence too her need to do his shirts and act in some measure in accordance with how a wife "ought to be." This wasn't just about delegating, this was about a belief system and her values apropos married life, and being a "good enough mother".

In the end a bit of creative reasoning on the part of her husband did the trick: he saw little point in her fulfilling varying chores because of some belief he wasn't even party to, and that her being less stressed because of extra time it afforded actually made him happier. Ditto in some respect her daughter who had begun to feel resentment at her mother's lack of trust.

This was hardly life shifting in terms of the amount of time it actually gave back to Rosy. But what she had done wasn't just about time, but rather about communicating her (very minimal) needs and entering into a collaboration with her family which turned a new corner. And while she was still choosing to have a couple of glasses of wine in the evening, it was now shared with her husband at an earlier time and without the bags of crisps.

Ask yourself:
Prioritizing...

Do you use food, snacking, picking during the day, to put off doing stuff or talking to certain people?

What in your day could you bring forward which would give you an immense sense of relief?

Delegating...

Is there anything, no matter how small, that you could let someone else do?

Do you have trust issues about letting people do things for you?

What would be the worst outcome if they didn't do the job as well as you would hope?

Would it matter?

Could you be gracious about it and let them learn on the job?

How might that person feel with the extra task or responsibility?

Can you check with them?

How would you feel if after a while you knew you no longer had to do whatever it is you'd be delegating?

Dump...

*What can you let **go** of?*

Does letting go make you feel anxious, even with something small?

Is there good reason for this?

If not, can you try letting go for a limited time, a day or a week?

Notice how you feel after the first week.

With all of the above, remember, less is more.. All that's needed initially is to find tiny **tipping points** which will lessen the stress or the emotion and the eating behaviour... often more than the sum of the parts. Notice any change in how you feel and subsequent eating behaviours. Notice the chain reaction!

Take note and collect the evidence!!

Prioritizing in action and time management:
The previous chapters will have highlighted much of the impact of time constraints and commitments on raising stress levels and their emotional knock on effect on eating patterns. It stands to reason that shifting any of this, however minimally, will help with that "chain reaction."

Another way of looking at how we can more effectively manage our time and what we are doing with it, is to look more closely at what we do on a daily basis. Whether this is a week day or a weekend, (which is relevant), think of how your day is spent from getting up in the morning to going to bed at night.

Depending on whether you are out at work or at home, (i.e. week day versus w/end), *make an hour by hour list from a.m. to p.m.* This shouldn't take longer than five minutes but again we are zooming in for a really close look which can help show where something incredibly small can be changed in some way.

-
-
-
-
-
-
-
-

Keeping to specifics think about:

What would you change, or change around?

-

What might you prioritize – if not already?

-

What might you dump?

-

Is anything missing?

-

Often there are chores we put off for one reason or another that drain our energy and worse, precipitate eating instead. If there is any part of your day where you are eating unnecessarily, this may be a huge clue!

Notice whether your eating behaviour is flagging up an alarm at any time.

-

-

-

-

-

-

Consider also:

What is within your control to change?

-

-

-

What is not?

-

-

When you make changes, whether it's shifting things around or letting them go entirely, notice whether your eating behaviour naturally moderates. Many overeaters ... overeat or pick when they are putting things off or feeling the pressure. The proof of the smallest change hitting the success button will soon show. Caroline Buchanan in her book "The

15 Minute Rule" explores exactly this and presents ways to overcome the inevitable resistance so we can get on with our lives (and not end up overeating!).

Remember, however small the success, it all adds up and begins to override the old habits.

As always, do the detective and collect the evidence! What, when, where, etc. and as ever...

Ask yourself:

What do I want? What am I willing to do? What am I able to do? What do I choose to do?

KEEPING IT SIMPLE:
LESS IS MORE FOR EFFECTIVE CHANGE...

Because things are rarely simple and the more people who rely on us, or whose timetables interconnect with our own, the more it becomes an issue to instigate change: because of this I really want to catch anyone this could relate to *before* the understandably jaded frustration sets in, and closes you down: often as not there is little head space or mental energy left, you may feel beyond exhaustion, and the only way you are functioning is on automatic, especially with comfort eating. You might be looking after children or an elderly parent, or your role might have shifted to being a part or full time carer depending on the level of care a person requires, and can be compounded by your emotional history together. I have met many, many carers whose weight escalated as their ability to go out and be "normal" was hampered by the need to be almost permanently present. Social services or respite care is usually only a few hours once or twice a week and by that time, going for a coffee and a cake and watching the world go by might be as much as you can muster.

Or you might have a child or a loved one in hospital. Apart from taking time off work, or adding to a working day if this is the case, the emotional exhaustion is often the bit that makes thinking out of the box almost impossible. Healthy eating out the window, more cake or hospital café food... etc etc...

So I am not going to pretend for a minute that any of what I suggest is going to make it all go away or wave some magic wand...

What I *am* going to suggest, as I did earlier, is that things are rarely a hundred per cent unchangeable. The tiniest of change which, if nothing else, might keep you hanging be it by the fingernails onto some semblance of sanity... might keep your eating patterns contained, and your escalating weight stable, till the cavalry arrives....

If you feel you can hardly operate let alone have energy to consider anything new, it *may* be that asking someone whose opinion you value could help provide fresh insight.

Joining a group can be a boon: many of the women especially, who were coming sometimes just for weight management for the kind of reasons I describe, would say that the couple of hours shared was their one bit of personal space and for being "normal".

One lady's only son had a heroin habit. Another person had come to the UK from the other side of the world with her husband and found subsequent to buying a house that he had advanced cancer. She struggled on her own to keep her job and make payments, whilst feeling emotionally at sea and without the support of family or friends nearby. The "small change" for each of these women was using the time in my weight management group simply to be with others, disclose whatever they felt would help them to be present and at least keep their eating patterns under some control. Sometimes just getting emotional space is the magic ingredient.

These are of course extreme situations and the irony is that less complicated lifestyles and circumstance don't necessarily mean we get any more of a handle on our eating behaviours. My intention is merely to reach out to anyone whose eating is spiralling out of control and say hey, you too!

* * *

Carrying on from the previous chapter the exercise here is to find the smallest thing which will make a difference. To do this needs yet again your detective skills and attention to detail, unearthing the smallest area for change, for maximum impact. The story I relate below demonstrates the potential impact of one such change.

Finding the Tipping Point...

One of my clients, Sally, is incredibly organized and because event planning is integral to her actual work she finds it easy, in principle, to manage her overeating by factoring shopping for food, cooking or eating out, into her schedule. In principle. She doesn't feel she overextends herself, but typically at some point in the month she gets overtired, overloaded, and while work plans are sacrosanct, the plans which affect her eating behaviours suffer in consequence.

Going through her day with almost microscopic attention to detail to find the key point at which something shifted in her managing her eating, what transpired somewhat unbelievably as the unwitting culprit was the washing up! Since much of Sally's life is a rush, coming home to a sufficiently welcoming home is hugely important. And "welcoming" for Sally, means tidy. A tidy enough home providing breathing space in an otherwise over full existence cluttered with never ending deadlines and targets. As needs must, she was able, skilfully, to prioritize on the run and park anything not immediately necessary to the side. The washing up however, though hardly crime of the century, was turning out to be a non negotiable: although Sally knew she hated it when overtiredness meant she left the dishes one day after the next, she had underestimated entirely just how much of a negative knock on effect it was having. Given the time to reflect it became clear that this was the moment when her eating behaviour, as if to provide a temporary stilling of the increasing upset on coming home to a mess, would become erratic and compulsive and get worse as the week went on.

Although her workload and too little sleep also factored in, the washing up was always the visible tipping point of the overload, and moreover, the easiest one to manage.

The holy grail question then, was whether Sally felt able and willing, now the knock on effect of that chain reaction was so much in evidence, to do the dreaded washing up at the very latest before leaving home each morning, and the more practical matter of whether a dishwasher might, if space in the kitchen, be a more than worthwhile investment under the circumstances! Motivated no doubt by the revelation as well as the ease with which this small effort might be managed, she was keen to "experiment" with immediate effect!

Despite that wonderful adage, "Be practical! Plan for a Miracle!" it would be foolhardy as well as naïve to expect an entire relationship with food to right itself after the tiniest of tweaks... but at least not for the want of not trying! Never say never! The purpose in this type of approach is to discover what triggers the overeating at its weakest point of leverage and experiment with change. Added to which, finding something relatively mundane and practical is quicker and less threatening than say, directly confronting your emotional issues, and may even lessen some of those emotional issues more than might be imagined.

Turning the telescope....

As I stipulate at the outset, calorie counting is not the full story. Turning the telescope away from the food and discovering what sets off the over eating, what triggers the cravings or the need for edible solace, is as key to the issue as what we actually eat. Again using the example of sleep deprivation, which reduces focus and heightens the desire for glucose or sugar or processed carbs...getting to bed early might be the challenge that needs working on rather than wondering day after day how come you just can't stop feeding!

Be innovative... Experiment!

Whatever you do, treat everything as an experiment: some ideas will turn out to be duds, but it's still information, and for our detective work – a process of elimination! Some ideas will work only some of the time, which is still great, and once in a while you'll discover a lottery win with a dynamic, more than the sum of the parts effect: a very small key to a life changing door!

Teasing out the triggers which are Tipping Points can be fun as well as insightful, and is all part of Doing the Detective. It lessens the tedium of dieting and makes your quest to create a better relationship with food so much more meaningful and that, my friend, is what we have to hold on to!

* * *

Harking back momentarily to my earlier mention of sharing with others..... It may neither be possible or even appealing to some people... but as well as offering practical assistance, finding a local support group can be intensely rewarding and help you feel less isolated if your eating habit is getting out of control. These groups are rarely "deep therapy" but *can* be deeply therapeutic and I list some of these at the back of the book.

For the road, I hope you like the piece of prose, on the value of sharing a journey. (I know, everything's a journey these days, but hey...) I came across it in Alaska many years ago, where the goose holds a place in mythology, and have always found it deeply moving.

THE SENSE OF A GOOSE

Author Unknown

In autumn, when you see geese heading south for the winter flying along in "V" formation, you might consider what science has discovered as to why they fly that way. As each bird flaps its wings, it creates an uplift for the bird immediately following. By flying in "V" formation, the whole flock has at least 71 per cent greater flying range than if each bird flew on its own.

People who share a common direction and sense of community can get where they are going more quickly and easily because they are travelling on the thrust of one another. When a goose falls out of formation, it suddenly feels the drag and resistance of trying to go it alone and quickly gets back into formation to take advantage of the lifting power of the bird in front. If we have as much sense as a goose, we will stay in formation with those people who are headed the same way we are.

When the head goose gets tired, it rotates back in the wing and another goose flies point. It is sensible to take turns doing demanding jobs, whether with people or with geese flying south.

Geese honk from behind to encourage those up front to keep up their speed. What message do we give when we honk from behind?

Finally, and this is important, when a goose gets sick or is wounded by gunshot and falls out of formation, two other geese fall out with that goose and follow it down to lend help and protection. They stay with the fallen goose until it is able to fly or until it dies; and only then do they launch out on their own or with another formation to catch up with their group. If we have the sense of a goose, we will stand by each other like that.

TRIGGER TRACKING…
making it Easy…

If your eating habit has become an overriding feature from getting up in the morning to going to bed at night, you possibly never feel hungry enough to notice what starts things off. It can seem as though we eat all the time and that everything is a trigger. Even minimally shifting your food intake however, and that can be quantity or content, (including fizzy drinks…) will have the effect of peeling away till at some point, you **will** find a **lead trigger** underneath the layers. This is always the one that gets the eating ball rolling in the first place, whether it's due to a time factor, a person, a situation, whatever, but ultimately this is the one that needs getting hold of in whichever way works best. Even plain old "habit" has its starting point: something set it off at the start and something holds it in place.

What "works best" may be a combination of strategy, enhanced motivation, and distraction. Whenever and wherever you can, finding other engaging distractions to lure you away from reoffending is the best way to mind that gap between your intention, and what you often end up doing. It's like you can have an argument with a child which can become a full blown tantrum, or you can take that child's hand and focus their attention on something more attractive. The Child, aka Monkey, or Pilot on Automatic, is that wee being within us who is intent on having the goodies and not the least bit interested in any counter rationale. So one has to be canny as well as loving. Think Jo Frost in Supernanny. She uses firm boundaries, but she also engages with the children in games that mean something to them. She has fun with them.

There can be an assortment of strategies but finding the tipping point, as with Sally earlier on, creates a foot in the door intervention: Sally's "foot in the door" was doing the washing up which used the knock on effect strategy in reverse: it had a positive impact on her eating behaviour without the direct tackling which can be counterproductive. Worth noting however that what actually came before this, was her **willingness** to look at what was going on for her. Over the page you will see an outline of Sally's original situation with its changed outcome once she'd put her foot in the door. The chain reaction was altered with minimal effort other than a willingness to be open and do something new.

What works best...

Rule Number One when looking for a tipping point and tackling any of these Triggers is to always, always start from what makes most sense to you, what's easiest to work with, for *you!!* It engages a process of ongoing achievement from the outset, and that is all that matters. Ultimately, my aim is that each person can become their own best "diet detective", their own best counsel, and that your knowing what's best for *you* will be as reliable as in areas where you are supremely confident.

It isn't about what might be easy for someone else but rather what works for you, so you *can* get your foot in the door. Wherever you are at, in a good place or not so great a place in your head, in or out of the zone as it were, start with something incredibly *easy*. Even though Sally felt the washing up ate into her personal downtime, once convinced at to its somewhat stunning effect, doing it was one hundred percent doable, as was the following example:

For many years I worked from home, and as I only had one living room, this was used for group work. This meant that a small second bedroom was used as an office for all other paperwork, and the predictable overflow from that, including my personal effects... would find themselves (note my abdication of responsibility... !) piled up on the double bed in my main bedroom. Let me make it clear that I am deeply aesthetically sensitive, and the mountain pile which grew over successive weeks left me feeling desperate and out of control, not to mention impacting my already bad record in getting enough sleep. Who after all would want to sleep in that?

I was working late into the evenings and at one point had just under ninety people coming a week, so it wasn't exactly laziness but my spiralling angst was reaching danger levels. Exhausted from lack of sleep and hateful at the sight of my room, I was having fantasies of running away from my own home (I *was* terribly tired..!!) till one day I spent eight hours tidying. I realise I sound like someone's belligerent teenage daughter but somehow I had attributed the extent of my despair onto other factors. The effect of the transformation was the mood equivalent of the door to Narnia! The veil of despair fell from me and I was renewed! Saul to Paul on the road to Damascus!

The point of this shaggy dog story is that this was not something I had to go out and pay for. Yes, as with Sally it did take an effort: I had a lot on and even if it was a terrible mess, it was an understandable mess. But once I appreciated just how badly it was affecting me, maintaining sufficient tidiness in my bedroom was no longer an option. Again, it was doable, even if the doing required effort. It was actually *easy:* moderate effort, maximum effect.

Using Easy to override old habits…

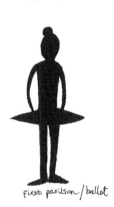

first position / ballet

Finding the least small thing each of you can do then, to restore the calm, or more pertinently your eating behaviours, to an acceptable state, is to find your personal *Easy!!!* Just like the first position in ballet, or the basic standing Tadasana / Mountain Pose in yoga, or your car in *park* mode, by returning always

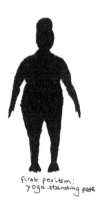

first position: yoga standing pose

to a position which you know, sets you straight, creates balance, restores order, and hence enables you to restart and continue from a point of success. Better still, it sets the precedent of installing a new habit to override the bad habits you've picked up and hardwired over time into your system. It may not always be directly food related but will absolutely have a direct bearing, down the line, on your Eating Behaviour. You will know this, because you will have seen it happen over and again, so you have evidence as opposed to simply a "felt" experience.

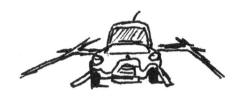

Car in "park" mode....

Reprogramming and Overriding the override:
The only thing you have to do is to find those Easy tasks and make it, or them, (as different ones may work for different situations), a new habit. Part of maintaining motivation over time, the bit that so many of us find so troublesome, involves both using overrides that have a fairly swift and positive result, (dieting already entails enough delayed gratification, so we need something here with a pretty swift reward factor!) and finding a way to *remind* ourselves. The beauty of habit as I reiterate over and again, is that like driving anywhere familiar, we can go into automatic, which means we need a pretty effective new habit to "override" the old. Which takes us back to wanting something enough, and an increasing amount of understanding and recognition.

It all takes time, but as with anything, the effort at the outset comes to life at some point and begins to fall into place. The detective work I'll be inviting you to do is to make a list of those *small but incredibly easy* tasks. They are like mini kick offs which get the motor started up and keep it going, in this case the motivation motor. And again, Montessori style, they are doable!

The *Easy* we have looked at here is a **Strategy**.

Later we'll look at *Easy* types of distraction and ways to engage your attention away from overeating and food... as in Lighting your Fire!

Restoring order in your life restores emotional breathing space... and pulls the eating behaviour out of spiral mode.

Sally's initial trigger situation

Over stressed and not dealing with workload well…

Peeling away the layers…

Sally's actual trigger situation

Dirty dishes everywhere

What I think	How I feel	What I end up doing…
Don't want to do them It's my free time…	Hate how it looks	Overeating, binging…

How it impacts another situation

Very stressed at work
Not managing well...
Snappy with colleagues…

What I think	How I feel	What I end up doing
I can't cope	Increasingly upset	Overeating even more

Foot in the door…

What I think	How I feel	What I end up doing
I need to change something	Open, willing, curious,	Doing the washing up at latest before leaving for work each day.

	How I feel now	What I end up doing
	Much happier, calm!	Eating normally

Detective work... following the crumbs...

Looking at the information you have collected so far, what chain reactions can you spot which end up with your overeating?

Testing it out:

What might be the smallest change you could put into place?

Collecting the evidence:

Make a note of what you believe could happen by making that change, then write down if it does happen.

Experiment:

It may not work every time, or at all, but you can experiment. It's a process of trial and error but will lead you to know what works best for you!

Always make a visible note of your evidence! We have a tendency to forget!

TURNING THE TIDE and restoring the balance...

Sometimes the tipping point may be less about stuff that needs to get done, and more about what gets overlooked: the non essentials we talk ourselves out of that put together, enable us to feel ok enough to keep going through the ups and downs, and ultimately, keep a lot of the stress related eating behaviours to a *minimum.*

Sometimes something transformational *is* what's required: it may be that a long overdue holiday *is* what you need to make the rest of your year even remotely workable.

That definitely needs including but I want to look first at things we put to the side which might take only *minutes,* yet get forever deferred in favour of what we believe is more important: we prioritize what *ought* to get done and what *should* get done, but discount in the process core needs which build up over time. Eventually, our urge to balance the equation, to restore some kind of balance, appears in our eating behaviours, small wonder. Leaving core needs unattended over time is like leaving a small child in a corner and wondering why they play up and start whining for attention. Or ignoring a strange noise in your car and wondering why it breaks down when you least need. Whichever analogy most hits the spot, the common denominator is neglecting areas of our life on the assumption they don't count and won't make so much of a difference. They do, and our overeating is frequently proof of that pudding.

Finding things which take minimal time means we are less likely to keep making excuses on the basis of *lack* of time. We are back once again to small, meaningful and easily achievable: minimal input for maximum effect.

Feeling overwhelmed by stress resulting from lack of time, lack of space, lack or excess of anything unpalatable… takes up a lot of head space: all too often our way to drown out or replace the horrible, space taking, time diminishing, stress induced scrunchy feeling, is by overeating, drinking, smoking, over spending… and any other manner of compensatory activities that come with a "cost to your health" tag. There is a correlating link to the behaviour which is by now adding as much upset to the entire equation as the original source of stress. Once again, we're back to those swinging metal balls and their chain reaction. And as we know with eating behaviours and weight, the cumulative, increasing knock on effect gradually reaches an exponential "Houston, we are *OUT* of control…!".

What you're looking for is anything which takes little time, helps you feel grounded and for a brief time at least, restores your sense of self amidst the mayhem. Very like pottering in the garden, doing a crossword or having time to read the paper. In essence giving yourself time to smell the roses, or in the words of W.H.Davies "time to stand and stare"[47]. No matter what, the feel good factor, which is the clue, will be quickly apparent: when we are drawn to something which engages us, it really is like a meditation: as our focus intensifies, the breathing slows and deepens, and we become still. Far from *taking* time, time seems to expand and the experience is space *creating*. It somehow puts a small area of sanctity, emotional and mental air to breathe, back into where it is most needed. It creates a *still point.*

---

[47] "Leisure" by W.H.Davies 1911.

It does *not* matter how inconsequential or apparently trivial whatever it is may seem to another person, though usually in these things, it is we who are our most merciless judges, pre-empting any statement with an apology, an attempt to explain "I know it seems stupid..." when the only "stupidity" would be not doing something which so easily restores equilibrium.

If knitting onesies or shining your car does it for you, that really is all that matters. The space in time you give yourself is at once magically multiplied, and minding that gap you might normally fill with eating. It's a *sabotage preventative* which helps you feel good and going back up the chain reaction - helps you stay slim. How good is that!!

Remember this is about doing something you enjoy on an immediately doable basis, which adds a more than the sum of the parts feeling of wellbeing to each day. Could be a walk in the park, fifteen minutes on your own at the beginning or end of the day, a half hour read, time to surf the net researching something you enjoy, whatever, but it lifts the spirit, and more significantly you frequently realise that for a brief duration, you have actually forgotten about food or eating. If you take ten or fifteen seconds imagining it, you may find yourself taking an unexpectedly deep breath as the body relaxes and calms.

Of *course* taking real time out for yourselves is ideal, but what I'm trying to convey here is the stuff you can do even without that much money or time, or perhaps even without that much physical and mental energy.

That then avoids the "Ah but..." conversation either with someone else, or inside your head. "Ah but I'm so busy, I'm too busy for my shirt..." to paraphrase Right Said Fred... is the bit that keeps your head buried in the sand and your eating behaviours unchanged.

As in...

...watching the sunrise / sunset......picking pebbles......morning tea......ten minutes downtime alone on coming home......a ten minute chat on coming home......a hug before you or your partner leaves for work......work of any particular kind......sharing with a friend......physical intimacy......a walk

round the park......being active......singing......with a choir......being with nature......an hour to read before bed......time to read the papers......learning an instrument......starting a new hobby......writing letters......

Ask yourself...

As you review your list, which you might be adding to regularly as the possibilities are endless, **how long** *and* **how often** *– daily, weekly etc do I need to do this to feel ok enough, enough of the time?*

-
-
-
-
-
-
-

What is the Tipping Point in terms of minimal time and frequency, for its effect to be felt?

- 15 minutes daily / twice a week / weekly
- 45 minutes twice a week...
- 90 minutes once a week... for example, a yoga class or choir...
-
-
-
-
-

- How often and how long starts to add up to a state of ***optimal wellbeing***.

My own example is that I feel a real sense of wellbeing when I have two giant mugs of tea every morning. I do not enjoy tea at any other time during the day, but this morning ritual, with time to reflect, is my sanctity. Such is the effect that when I am not able to have this, something feels at odds with my day which I am likely to placate later on with unnecessary food. Such is the value I place on this, that while obviously, in an emergency such as the house being on fire and my backside being alight, I may have to give it a miss, I have factored in an extra hour even when my flights were at 4 in the morning, and even with the die hard yoga training I did for six weeks some years ago entailed yet again a 4am rise. (My German room mate wasn't so taken by this, but I felt her cleaning her teeth with such unnecessary vigour at a late hour in the adjoining en suite each night, rather evened the odds.)

Here are some examples people have given…

WELLBEING LIST:

Go swimming once a week

Have fifteen minutes on own before family / kids get up

Leave work ON time to have an hour extra with kids / family

Purchase the particular brand of coffee / tea etc that I love best and savour!

Get off one station earlier to walk through the park to go to work.

Do fifteen minutes Pilates every day

Phone at least one friend a week for half an hour

Watch a favourite programme a couple of times a week, rather than giving in to everyone else…

Allow time to read the papers on Sundays…

* * *

MINDING the GAP and WINDOWS of TIME...

One of the other reasons for finding outlets or stress busters that take a minimal amount of time, and can be fitted in with some degree of flexibility – is that when one of those eating urges arises, (and I do not mean when you are genuinely hungry) there is often a window of time that they last, if we are able to distract ourselves for the duration. Particularly if we have fixated on a food item, such as a now open bar of chocolate, willpower alone rarely works, and it's more a case of *when* rather than *if* we will finally succumb. It's why, other than the need for a level of resolve and putting boundaries in place which pre-empt the urge, (if you haven't purchased the item, it isn't there...) your base level of motivation is given a huge helping hand with distractions which you've already thought about and prepared for.

So this time, make a list of anything and everything which could simply serve as a distraction. Even if you can't think of anything off the top of your head, keep your eyes and ears and heart and body open for noticing, be it after the fact, anything seemingly small in effort which has that taking you away from the focus of feeding effect...!

as in...

Manicuring nails etc

Abdominal crunches using the floor while watching the news...!

Cleaning, filing, reading a magazine ...

Your own...

-
-
-
-
-
-
-

TIP: If some of the task related tipping points from the previous chapter have the same effect, include these in your list. I once had a flatmate who said when she did her weekly ironing, it gave her the sense that all was right in the world and restored her feeling of order and calm. All you want is anything which has a distracting, stilling effect and lessens emotionally reactive eating.

The focus is on the *quality* of the effect on you, and your eating behaviour, rather than what you are actually doing.

LIGHTING YOUR FIRE
and other distractions...

LIGHTING YOUR FIRE
and other distractions…

Turning the Tide looked at time efficient ways of grabbing your attention, taking your mind off food, calming stress levels, and generally tipping that knock on effect back in the right direction.

LIGHTING YOUR FIRE turns up the volume and is about anything which fills you with **passion** and adds **meaning** and **purpose** to your life:

It *may* only be ten or fifteen minutes a day, it may be more, but it is far more than a mere distraction: whatever it is… is deeply engaging; it holds you and contains you and nourishes you. Over time, it can be subtly transformational. It provides a stimulus that engages the senses, and when becoming part of the fabric of your regular life, it provides a certain structure. If you look back to your relationship with food, something which "lights your fire" offers, extraordinarily, much of the same but without the "codependence". It might be something you **do,** it might be people you spend time with, it might simply be a way of being or now that there is such incredible travel choice, it might be time spent away with a difference. In short, whatever the "it", it *feeds* a part of ourselves we often dismiss as unimportant.

Nourishing and feeding the soul…

When we have something which **lights our fire** it fills a gap all too frequently filled with food. Eating provides stimulus and structure and meaning to our lives. **Over**eating is often an attempt to carry this further which would be fine if it were not at a cost. Often what we need is **chicken soup for the soul**: its nourishment is authentic and far more enduring.

One lady, Jan, whose addiction to food was so extreme it was almost all she gave thought to every day, whether battling against her urge or giving into it, found her only respite was whenever she spent time in the wild: she first noticed this during a fortnight whale watching somewhere off South Africa's Cape Town coast, when she described herself as being "so captivated" that she "forgot" her usual preoccupation. Another time although less dramatic, a working holiday on a farm produced a similar freeing from what she called her " inner torture".

Helen, another client, rented a mobile home for a year after her divorce. I cannot now recall why she didn't carry on with this apparently idyllic sojourn, especially as she had work nearby, but during that year she found that along with feeling calmer and more at peace than ever before, her tendency to binge, frequently, had remarkably abated: as she reverted to regular, healthy eating which she enjoyed, the weight fell off with little apparent effort.

These stories are as noteworthy as they are inspirational, and I cannot help but suspect that their extreme overeating, in the light of its sudden cessation with changed circumstances, was that old "red warning light" which we ignore at our peril. Each of them were relatively free of the familial and financial restrictions that keep many of us bound to the tether, so I wondered, privately at the time, what kept them stuck with so much possibility for change, and their health at stake...The Monkey Story at the end of this chapter provides a refreshing take on exactly this question.

S.O.S... Saving our Souls... Stimulating our Senses!!!
Needless to say, most of us have obligations and commitments and cannot go wafting off on some Ecuadorian gap year to "find ourselves", without seriously rocking the boat!

What we can do in the interim however, are mini versions of the same. We can weave things into our lives that fill our hearts. I'm looking more at emotionally driven eating here, since someone whose family and children fills their hearts may be overeating because of food and cooking being such a heavy part of the equation! This is a little different!

What I am suggesting is to begin noticing *anything* you do which lifts your spirit so much that even for a short while, you are lost in time, and forget your usual preoccupation with food. When we are engaged, transfixed almost with something which feels good, it is as though we enter a point of **stillness.** It doesn't need filling... because it *is* fulfilling.

248

The **Still Point,** to quote T.S. Eliot[48] is where the dance **is...**

It *may* be that your life needs to change dramatically and that excessive overeating (or drinking or smoking for that matter) is a red warning sign that something within is out of synch. Out of harmony.

Or it may be that your life needs just a bit of subtle alteration to achieve a better balance.

Jot down a list of anything you think of which as it comes to mind, has a momentary stilling, or uplifting effect. Anything you enjoy which you could easily give more time to...

YOUR LIST:
Mundane to magical, it all counts:

-

-

-

-

-

-

-

Put this list somewhere you can see and add to it over the days and the weeks. See if you can even feel a sense of positive **anticipation** as you collect ideas, and then, where possible, put them into action. The beauty of our eating behaviours is that they are so easy to spot when they occasionally, almost magically, moderate. So **experiment!** Once again, this is your detective in action!

Notice too, anything you do that makes you feel good, grounds you, brings you back to a sense of peace and right*ness*. Brings a sense of order

---

[48] T.S.Eliot's The Still Point: Burnt Norton 1936. Subsequently part of The Four Quartets 1943.

which enables you to recharge. Which of these things are essential to your wellbeing?

Remember it *could* be getting up early enough to watch a sunrise, or it could be putting your many years of photographs into an album, whether digital or hard copy! It might be taking up a labour's love of tapestry, or "American quilt making" filled with bits of material from years of sentimental remnants, or it might be taking time to paint a picture.

One of my clients would describe how her love of photography took her to "another world" within herself, while another took to knitting colourful scarves and sometimes more intricate jumpers to help stop her snacking. In each case, whether it's your daily crossword or frankly even arranging pebbles in a garden, whatever it is becomes more of a ***ritual...*** which helps ***override the ritual of overeating...***

Tip: It can be quite challenging to begin something at the end of a week day when we are often just that bit too drained to initiate anything new. If this is the case and what you are going to experiment with is just a little more adventurous or initially time consuming, you might want to make inroads on a weekend, or when you do indeed have some time to spare. If this is the case though, make sure you set a time frame!!! That way, like Blue Peter of old, when you come home at night or have your first bit of spare time later in the evening, you can bring out "something you prepared earlier!!"

Tip: Remember the exciting bit, other than just getting going with something you enjoy... is noticing how your eating *moderates*. Ok, without actually watching the kettle boil, but over time, collect the evidence!!

Along these lines.....

What do you talk yourself out of?

-

-

-

For optimal wellbeing, what do you love to do / go to, etc?

-

-

How long do you need to do it to feel sufficiently sane, to operate on a daily level at your best, for optimal performance?

-

-

How often do you need to do it?

-

-

Which of these mean the most to you?

-

-

-

How many of these do you do already or need to do more of?

-

-

What could you put in place this week?

-

-

This month?

-

-

This year?

-

-

MINDING THE GAP: LIFE BALANCE CHECK…

Overeating then is often a way to try to restore the balance, to placate emotionally and to fill the unfulfilled, and were it not for the weight and ensuing health implications, it would be more than fit for purpose and do a rather wonderful job. There may be a conscious awareness of a sense of imbalance, or it might be unrecognised, and it need not be all consuming, but as we know, even small, chronic longings and irritations have a way of building up over the years.

Reviewing your current lifestyle, how much time do you spend on various areas in your life such as relationship / family / work / recreation / social / chores / paperwork / health / other…?

Think about what these areas mean to you. For example, your work and recreation might be one and the same, or to you, work might equal "chores" or "paperwork". Equally, if you've been married for a decade or more, family may mean something different to "relationship", which in turn will be different if you've just begun dating.

Have a look at the example below then divide the circle overleaf to reflect this, but do have fun with it! (You may prefer to do separate ones for weekdays and weekends.) It isn't schoolwork and there isn't a "right way". It's about how *you* feel things pan out. So, taking into consideration the most important areas of your life, fill the circle so that each portion is representative of how much of your time, or your energy, it takes up.

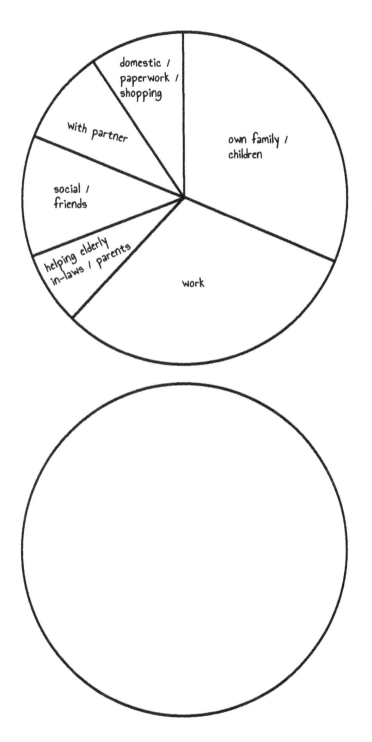

You might want to think a little out of the box:

- A social worker whose workload stayed in her head long after leaving, drew a far larger pie chart percentage than her actual working hours.

- Similarly, a teacher whose 9 to 5 hours barely reflected work taken home over so many years.

- Another lady whose fluctuating shifts badly affected her sleep, also drew a larger percentage than the actual hours she worked.

Looking at your circle, are you content with the balance or the division of your life as it is reflected, or does it show where certain areas take up too much or too little time?

*What might be **missing?***

-

-

-

-

-

*What you might like to have **less** of?*

-

-

-

-

*What you might like to have **more** of?*

-

-

-

-

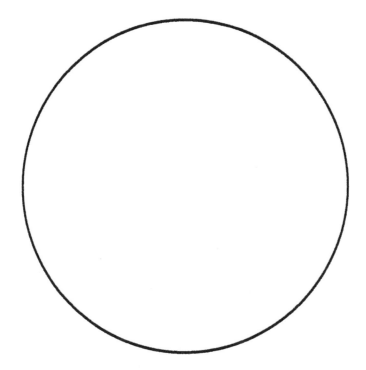

When you have thought about this, draw another circle and this time re-jig it so that each portion represents the balance you would **prefer** to have or includes what might have been **missing**. How would it look if you were to spend the time you want or need in given areas of your life?

Notice:

What are the areas of difference?

-

What might you do to redress the balance?

-

What are the current priorities in your life?

-

Does this match the time you give it in a day?

-

Do some areas take more time than you would wish and detract from more preferable areas? (This may seem insignificant but over a life time, adds up.)

-

What changes could you make to have a more balanced lifestyle? Don't forget, it's your idea of "balance", not someone else's.

-

How could you do this?

-

Where do you feel you have little choice?

-

Where possibly do you abdicate responsibility – blaming it on outside circumstance or another, when in fact it is you stopping yourself?

-

-

-

Ask yourself, what is it that stops you, if anything?

-

-

-

Again, the shift worker included a massive portion for *sleep* and stipulated a need for at least seven hours for several consecutive nights! An interesting inclusion as most people would take this for granted.

- The teacher and the social worker wanted more quality time with family and friends. Both also drew in their second circle a much larger slice for personal time.

- An office worker drew in time for going outdoors and being active.

It's not about having to make radical changes, though for the record, the social worker did eventually change career completely as the correlation with overeating became so overwhelming: it's about increasing your awareness, so that even if it becomes evident that life changing moves might be hugely beneficial, or even imperative at some point in the future, you can *choose* to make the small changes or additions we've been looking at, *here and now.*

And again, think *outside of the box* when you can, as well as heeding your intuition: it's about doing (or not doing) something which not only serves a purpose, but alleviates the eating behaviour activity at the end of the chain reaction!

If for example, you long for physical contact and you're lucky enough to live somewhere relatively urban – there are wonderful Cuban Ruedo, Mirenge, Salsa and ballroom dance classes *and* workshops out there now, that provide male dance partners for the over abundance of single women, (even for the seriously left footed) and these are *not* all leg over joints, (unless it's just me being given a wide berth…!). Ditto a wealth of tango clubs have sprouted countrywide.

If you work from home or for whatever reason, your social life has reduced to zilch, there are great "Meet Ups" around the country with different interests which can be found from the internet.

It *may* not replace what you believe you need, like for like. But it fills something in a way other than over eating. It *may* not be everything you want, but could be a lot of what you need. And if you can remotely convince yourself there's no link with eating behaviours, test it out. Experiment and record your eating behaviour results on a daily basis. Collect the evidence.

Remember we often overeat when we need better sleep, when we have too much or too little to do. We overeat to entertain ourselves and create a stimulus, and we overeat when something more vital is lacking.

We may not be able to make up exactly for the lack, but it is a pointer. Emotionally reactive eating always serves a function, or rather mis-serves it, but it points to where the gap lies. It points to where our need for something more meaningful or where our need for healing, might lie.

"We all need something to do,
Somewhere to live,
Someone to love…"

(Adapted from Erik Erikson's Stages of Psychosocial Development….!)

MINDING THE GAP: FULFILLING YOUR POTENTIAL

Many of the gaps in our lives, our daily existence, are on the mundane level. It doesn't lessen their impact but none the less they may revolve around a need for distraction, whether that is social or professional or personal, and eating all too often fills that gap. On a deeper level, that gap can be the search for something of greater meaning which perhaps evades us, or is for some reason out of reach. It is one that relates much more to *who* we are and *why* we are here. It is far more to do with a sense of purpose and fulfilling potential[49].

For some people this is less demanding but for others, the unmet call to do or become something which has greater meaning can create the most powerful discontent[50]. If you eat to block out or to quell emotion, no prizes here for what ends up happening.

Remembering that emotions tell us something, provide valuable information, if this describes you in any way, ask yourself when the negative feelings most arise? What might they relate to?

-

-

-

Ask yourself:

When am I happiest?

-

-

What fills me with passion? Or longing?

-

-

---

[49] Caroline Myss Sacred Contracts: Awakening your Divine Potential. Bantam Books 2001. www.myss.com
[50] Nathaniel Branden Honouring the Self: Self-Esteem and Personal Transformation. Bantam Books 1983 www.nathanielbranden.com

When do I feel life is most meaningful?

-

-

If time or money or commitments prevent personal fulfilment in some way, what would I do if this were not the case?

-

-

-

If I could live again, what would I do differently?

-

-

What might I most regret if left unfulfilled?

-

-

Then:

What would you do right now, if you could?

-

-

What are your main priorities in life?

-

-

Are you doing any of these at the moment?

-

-

If not, why not? What stops you?

-

-

What practical things might you put in place, within the next week or month, to honour some of these?

-

-

Consider whether any of this affects your eating in any way?

-

-

When you *are* honouring whatever your priorities are, that inner calling, do you find you eat more moderately? Begin to notice this over time.

The psychiatrist, Carl Jung, said that to be whole and healthy, we need to heed what calls from within. This is not some mysterious voice but usually arises as a natural instinct. It usually makes itself felt wherever we find joy in being a particular way, or following a particular path, or interest. As you read the following story, listen to your heart and write down any thoughts or feelings.

THE MONKEY STORY
Or THE ILLUSION of FREEDOM

In some countries, to catch a monkey, they put food (of monkeyish appeal) into a stone or granite container with a hole, just large enough for the monkey's hand to slip through and grasp. Problem for the monkey being that once his little paw is tightly clenched around what he so longs to have, the widened shape of his fist can't be retracted from the heavy stone.

He can't escape – but he doesn't think to let go. He is stuck. And as his captors approach he is seemingly ensnared in a situation from which he believes there is no escape. Apparently...

... sound familiar? Ring any bells?
What things, thoughts or beliefs
> *Do you hold onto*
>> *Which seem absolutely fixed or essential...*
>>> *But*
Prevent you from living a life of greater freedom?
Where or how, with whom or with what,
> *Do you feel most stuck,*
>> *Unable to let go?*
If your memory needs jogging, think about that lifestyle, relationship or habit you can barely afford, be it emotionally or financially, or physically.
Is your relationship with food in any way like this?
Where is your "paw" so tightly clasped that your freedom is curtailed?
What do you talk yourself out of...
> *... that really isn't an option*
>> *in terms of physical, emotional*
>>> *and spiritual wellbeing?*
What stops you?
Does this affect your eating behaviour in any way?
If you were not afraid, what would you be doing?

There will be people who *know* what they would love to have done, been, be doing, but are either afraid, or feel circumstances make it impossible, in which case the story above can offer, at the least, an interesting perspective!

On the other hand there are many people who know they would like to do more with their lives, and please bear in mind this does not have to be academic or professional, but somehow can't pin it down to any one thing.

Especially for the latter, have a dip into the reading below. There are a thousand and one books on the subject, but these are a great take for anyone whose path is very unclear, or a bit off the beaten track.

Over and above this, there are wonderful workshops out there which may or may not pertain directly to "your calling", yet have a natural effect on opening us up to our true or distantly buried selves! (See Appendix)

Anything which is going to simultaneously moderate the compensatory overeating, *and* have fun at the same time, can't be bad, surely!

It's never too late to become the person you might have been!

George Elliot

PART 4:
DISTORTED THINKING AND HOW WE SEE THINGS

HOW WE SEE THINGS...
and other beliefs and assumptions...

Back in the '90s The Guardian ran a TV advert that opened with a young, muscular, shaven headed guy covered in tattoos and piercings, who suddenly began running down a street. The camera then swung to a bespectacled, middle aged gentleman in a suit holding a brief case, waiting for a bus. He saw the first man and started to look uncomfortable. As the tattooed guy began gaining speed, the "city gent" clutching his case ever tighter with a look of increasing alarm, the camera continued to shoot to and fro till the other, a yard or so away... lunged toward him...

The picture then froze for a few seconds with the first chap mid-air. What do you think was about to happen?

The next shot is a still of the man at the bus stop. At this point the camera zooms back allowing a much wider view, and what we see is a pile of scaffolding that is collapsing and close to crushing him. The person who had seen this happening, who for all intents and purposes many of us thought was "a thug", lunges and pushes him out of the way, a second before the scaffolding crashes onto where the older man had been standing.

Surprised? For most of us the revelation of what was actually going on was counterintuitive to presuppositions made on the basis of a limited vision and assumption of "type". The point however, was a brilliant advertising campaign for the newspaper which then flashed its slogan "...We give you the *full picture*..." and demonstrable proof of the speed with which we make judgements on either too little information, or because we have made an assumption.

Much of what we believe and take for granted about the world and ourselves will affect how we see things: how we see things will be enormously influenced by how we were brought up, the beliefs and assumptions of our family, our peers, our community, our culture, our generation, our education, our country, our ethnicity, our social status, and all that myriad of circumstances which conspire to create our sense of who we are within that world. Our entire belief system – is as much a part of the context – as things which are tangible and visible and right before our eyes. The difference is that it alters how we perceive and interpret a situation, and this usually has more relevance in terms of outcome, than the situation itself. Our history too, collective as well as personal, creates much of our perceptual framework. Where this is problematic is when these beliefs are detrimental, and cast an equally long shadow over our future, causing unnecessary suffering in the process. Often then, the tapestry of our past becomes interwoven into our physical, emotional and psychological make-up, and our bodies as well as our minds reflect this toll upon our wellbeing.

So what has this to do with overeating?

Our perception of **anything** affects how we think and feel, and ultimately how we behave. If your relationship with food is largely emotionally driven, then your eating behaviour may be a knock on effect from any experience which underlies those emotions.

> *PERCEPTION of an event will influence our ATTITUDE, our*
> *THOUGHTS, our FEELINGS and hence our BEHAVIOUR.*

Put another way, it isn't just a situation in itself that creates an outcome, but our reaction to it:

> *EVENT + RESPONSE = OUTCOME*

If that outcome is all too often an overuse of food to compensate, we need first to get wise to it, second, to check out our version of events and whether there might be an alternative viewpoint, and if we are indeed correct, then third, to see if we can change our response.

As a weight management counsellor, where I have seen this most visibly in action over the years is when people come to get weighed.

Many of you will have had this experience. Prior to getting on the scales and especially if it is a weekly event or after a long break, your anticipation is likely to fall somewhere between excitement and dread, with "ok enough" being the middle range. Whilst I have marvelled (and shared) the elation that even a small loss in the right direction can bring, I have witnessed as frequently the exact opposite to what has often been a mere minimal gain. The visible mood shift when a person neither expected, nor believed they *deserved* to have x lbs extra, is proof of perception in action: worse, the frequency with which this then has a knock on effect on a person's eating behaviour is the main concern. It is beyond easy to understand that when great effort has been made to regulate eating, an outcome in the wrong direction is hugely demoralising, and all too typically continued overeating is a reaction to frustration or upset. There's a perverse logic which says "Oh heck! What's the point! I may as well....." etc etc...

What is easily forgotten is that many things contribute to weight gain such as hormonal fluid retention, fluid retention due to illness, and sometimes fluid retention due to humidity, intense heat, or even being at altitude. Equally – watching the kettle boil – as I call it when a person is overly focussed on moment to moment weight loss, does not allow for bodily variations throughout a week or a month. Or indeed a momentary lapse.

One client many years ago with serious overeating issues, described herself as stoically pragmatic and said that if ever she made one mistake, that would be it. (My response *now* to such a statement would be to encourage a person to explore its implications before continuing, but this was early in my career and I suspect I did not do this sufficiently at the time.) Hence she proceeded valiantly in controlling her eating for five months, losing five stone in the process, till tired and upset one day she had a bad lapse. When she came to the group that week and discovered she'd gained seven pounds she remained true to her word and said she wouldn't be returning. Despite our attempts to reach her and connect with her in some way, and despite her staying for the duration offering a glimmer of hope, this lady chose to honour a non serving value - "one mistake equals failure" - over and above the evidence of her months of success.

Because that is *exactly* what is happening when we let a long running belief, or script[51], take precedence when it no longer holds true, nor serves us in any way. Many people for example will have a concept of failure

---

[51] Eric Berne "Games People Play: The Psychology of Human Relationships" Penguin Group 1964.

which diminishes everything they touch, yet a different outcome is not always failure: it is simply a different outcome. One mistake does not blot the whole copy book. But a long lasting reaction can do exactly that. Eating issues apart, negative emotions such as regret or anger can cast a far longer shadow into our future lives than the originating events.

Thinking back to our TV advert, it is always worth asking yourself:

Am I seeing the *whole* picture, or is my focus fixed on one small but miserable *corner* of the picture?

When a person says they are completely depressed, or their lives are terrible, does this mean they are depressed 24/7, without a *glimmer* of light? Does this mean that their *whole* life is without respite, hope, or anything good, or have they become stuck in an overly bad *slice section* of experience?

Ditto the entire dieting process: success is not about managing your eating regime, whatever that maybe, without fault. Success is the ability to get right back and carry on in as balanced a frame of mind as you are able. Which means less of the self recrimination which, as I reiterate, serves to no avail whatsoever.

whole experience...

the full picture...

XX < current negative perspective

Changing a reaction to something might indeed be a work in progress, but it's always going to be a whole lot easier if we are able to see a different viewpoint, or if additional information comes into play.

Can you think of any situations which directly, or indirectly, have an effect which end up with you overeating? Think of one or two recent examples.

-

-

-

In each case, do you believe you have the **full picture** or might new information provide an alternative way of seeing things?

Ask yourself:

What is the assumption you have made?

-

-

What is the evidence?

-

-

If true, is it true:

All of the time;

Some of the time;

Only once in a while;

-

-

If the assumption is correct a lot of the time, what does that mean?

What do you feel it says about you?

-

Do you need to overeat to comfort yourself, or can you catch yourself beforehand and do something different?

-

Benefit of insight...

One client, Helen, would find her apprehension rising disproportionately whenever her supervisor commended her for work well done. She would spend the whole day eating biscuits in a state of upset and imagining the worst. When I asked her how come a compliment made her so anxious, it transpired that in her last job, some years before, she had been praised but later on lost a promotion because she had "failed to keep up with expectations".

The "evidence" was that in her current job she had done well and had worked her way up based on merit. She feared however, that she had reached as far as she could go and that history would repeat itself. Yet with thought she realised she was in fact happy with her work, and didn't feel the need to fight her way further up the ladder; that she could maybe accept the positive comments on face value… and had no need to worry. On reflection though, she decided to request a review with her supervisor to allay a concern that her anxiety might indeed be picking up on something behind the scenes.

What was doubly beneficial was that the process of addressing her concerns not only took her from a place of vulnerability and anxious imaginings to one of strength and certainty, but impressed her supervisor with her ability to take charge. The most noticeable effect though was her return to normal eating!

Reality check...

Another client, Kathy, would find herself upset and infuriated by her mother-in-law's comments about aspects of her domestic competence whenever she visited. Her husband's shirts were never as white as they could be, the pastry a little heavy, her management of money apparently wanting for improvement and so on.

I imagine many of us would find the remarks... grating... but the assumption behind it was that mother-in-law didn't think she was good enough for her son. Although to try and keep the peace for the sake of her husband, Kathy wouldn't respond, her upset still shifted her mood, (not surprisingly really!) and in "sitting" on what she was tempted to say, would "eat her words" and end up overeating instead. The overeating would then continue throughout the week.

Fortunately... having been able to offload some of her upset in the group and realising that her "felt sense" of being not good enough was perhaps more down to her own insecurities, Kathy took advantage of time alone with her mother-in-law a few weeks later to tell her as gently as she could, that the criticisms left her feeling hurt and unvalued. To her amazement, she (the mother-in-law!) disclosed that she had feared being forgotten, and felt in some perverse act of logic that by pointing out the domestic shortcomings, it might make her son appreciate her all the more, when it was actually having the opposite effect.

I say fortunately because human interaction is rife with complexity and dynamics: it can be incredibly difficult to speak gently, as Kathy did, if what we are upset about has roots going way back in family history, and someone's reaction is defensive rather than open and amenable. Similarly if your work environment is toxic, and the "assumption" that openness would elicit reprisals, or lose your job, has good ground, a rule of thumb would be to keep to the facts, keep to the present time, and never use words like never!

There may well be times when we might ask ourselves, does it *really* matter, and choose to let something ride. Where we might **choose** otherwise however, is when the cost to our wellbeing is at stake as with overeating, and an increased risk to health. There's not much point letting something "ride" if you're not actually letting it **go!**

Although Kathy's overeating was hardly all due to her upset in this example, it was having a detrimental effect on her efforts to stabilise her eating habits, and so her weight, along with her blood pressure, had begun going back up.

Additionally, as with Helen, the step she took in addressing her mother-in-law and her success in managing this with care and respect, empowered her considerably.

Taking ourselves out of a defensive, or potentially victim like position to one of strength is as enabling as it is mature.

Whilst we may not always choose, or for that matter feel able, to act with such level headed maturity, (!), an escalating negative reaction impacting your relationship with food may be the deciding factor.

In this case, the steps below may help toward a positive outcome!

Caution:

- Keep any grievances to the one in question. Be clear about the behaviour which is affecting you and stick to the facts.

- In other words keep to the present time: the *here and now*.

- Be clear with yourself *before* the fact about the outcome you'd prefer. What do you *want?*

- Do not assign blame but stick to how their *behaviour* makes you *feel*.

- State what you would *prefer* them to do or say.

- When you have a conversation make sure the person you are speaking with is fully present and is able to pay attention and *hear* you.

- *Never...* use words like "you always / never..." etc. Its implication goes too far back in time and is usually incendiary.

- If you feel over emotional, whatever you do, *wait*. Do *not* strike while the iron is hot.

- If you feel likely to blow, ask yourself "What will it *serve?*"

I am not remotely suggesting this is a walk on the beach. If you know however, that you are unlikely to remain calm and collected and unblaming, however understandable, and however much nine out of ten of us would agree, you might want to decide before the fact whether it will be worth it. Once in a while, it is. Once in a while, the irrevocable is our redemption, but more often than not it crosses a line and is damaging, at the very least, to your eating behaviours at the end of that chain reaction.

In amongst the sentences below are a few platitudes. I am not a great fan of platitudes, but if one or two hit the spot, I can live with them. Have a look and maybe make up a few of your own:

Don't let one bad day ruin an entire journey.

Don't let one blot ruin the copy book.

Don't be trapped by a point of view.

Don't be held to ransom by what seems like a virtue.

An isolated incident does not a failure make!!

Success... in weight holding terms is about overriding knee jerk, all or nothing reactions.

Success... is the ability to bounce back. It is about resilience and balance.

Do... focus on what you've done well.

Do ... look at the whole picture.

Context might be everything, but ask yourself always:

- Might there be a different way to see something?

- Is there any way I might see this differently?

- How might that affect the outcome?

THINGS WE TELL OURSELVES...

Sometimes our perception of something is at fault because we lack information. That information might be the other person's perspective, as with Kathy's mother-in-law, it might be factual information which is needed, or it might be the lack of information that comes with experience. Sometimes however, our own history colours our ability to see things clearly. Even when we are sure we know our own minds, a lot of the fundamental strands to our belief system are not easy to see, especially when they relate to core beliefs about[52] ourselves.

---

[52] Christina Padesky: Constructing New Core Beliefs: A CBT Master Class (UK) 2013 www.padesky.com

Core beliefs, as they are often called, are those thoughts and ideas we have taken on board from others around us such as family, culture etc. They can be positive, neutral or negative, and like stereotyping or prejudice, they may or may not be accurate or even true. They are beliefs we have "swallowed whole" to the extent that we barely realise, let alone question, and probably act on the basis that they are factual. They are like seeds that have been sown long before we were able to think, or work things out for ourselves, and whilst some of them may stand us in good stead, others may not operate in our best interests. It is those beliefs which often most defy any rationale, (from an adult or intellectual perspective), and yet silently and resiliently pervade our lives and keep us in bondage, that most need tracing, tracking, and uprooting…!!

Even assuming a level of self awareness and maturity, when the chips are down or we are tired and miserable, these beliefs can pop up scarily from under the floorboards at a moment's notice.

Here's what a load of them look like:

Blanket statements about ourselves:
I'm unlovable
I'm hateful
I'm bad / crap / rubbish
I let people down
I'm useless
I'm a loser
I'm stupid
I'm hopeless
I'm unworthy
I can't change
I'm unacceptable
I'm a disappointment
I'm a failure
I always mess up
I'm ugly
I'm boring

Add your own ...!

-

-

-

-

Blanket statements about others and the world in which we live:
People don't like me
Things will never get better
Life is crap
Men / women are liars
Women are gold diggers
Men are bastards
Love is for fools
You can't trust people
People lie
People always disappoint me
No one trusts me

Add your own...!

-

-

-

-

The thing to remember here is that even assuming you are aware of a negative belief somewhere beneath the layers... even if you know full well, rationally, that it isn't true, it can still *feel* true. That's why it's important to keep adding to your list of when the opposite is true. ***Collect the evidence!!***

Once you start to notice its existence, or if overeating alerts you to their existence, question it:

Ask yourself:

Is this true?

What is the evidence?

Is it true some of the time, or all of the time?

If it is true, what does that mean about you?

*Can you think of times when it is **not** true, or when the opposite is true?*

Would someone you value see it the same way, or might they have a different perspective?

Say to yourself:

*Even though I might **feel** this way, that doesn't make it true.*

*Even though I might feel this way some of the time, it doesn't make it true **all** of the time.*

*Even though I **feel** like a failure at the moment doesn't mean I **am** a failure.*

*Even though I **feel** unlovable (e.g. because my partner's just left me) doesn't mean I **am** unlovable.*

We often turn one offs into absolutes. So for example, your partner leaving may certainly make you feel unloved, by that person, but it doesn't mean you *are* unlovable.

In the same way as I caution against using the "you always / you never" accusation with others, as it usually has an undesirable effect, be wary similarly of using it with yourself:

I.e. it may be true that you are a failure / unlovable / bad… **some** of the time, but it's unlikely this is all of the time.

It is very, very easy to selectively focus on the negative, both with ourselves and others. But ask yourself, is this the *full* picture?

-

*Are there instances when the negative belief is **not** true?*

-

If for example, you are feeling a failure, make a list of the many times you have been "a success". Think across the board, not just professionally or academically:

One morbidly obese client who deeply regretted never resuming a career she'd dropped to have children and be a stay at home mother, said she felt "her whole life was an utter failure".

Whilst her intensity of regret was undeniable, this same person had also casually mentioned on a different occasion that her three children, now grown up, had each said what a wonderful mother she was, and how grateful they were for their upbringing!

No mean accolade as any parent will know, so whilst not undermining the reality of part of her life being unlived, the *full picture* offered another perspective: it was not true that her entire life had been an utter failure. Far from it. A very key part of it was missing, unrealised, but its colouring her entire perspective was neither true nor helpful. Acknowledging that, from her own children's perspective, the part of her life she had chosen to pursue, be it at a cost, had in fact been profoundly successful, was *enabling.*

Additionally, remembering that she had made a choice, and one that had worked out supremely for three particular individuals, was equally enabling.

Widening the perspective to allow a "fuller picture" also helped Mary recognise that the time was ripe to explore new outlets for her considerable creative energy: the intensity of her now relentless regret, and the eating which seemed to accompany it, was demanding attention. The red warning light was flashing insistently!

Recognising that a negative belief is *not* the whole truth, is not the case all of the time, and is only part of the picture, may result occasionally in an instantaneous shift: a viscerally felt moment of release that frees us from the old reaction... and the eating habits that compensate.

More usually however, it is a gradual process. It may take tenacity and persistence to keep saying to ourselves, "just because I feel this way, does not make it fact". It may take perseverance to keep collecting proof to the contrary. But that is what you must do.

Reality check:
If your negative feeling is about something specific, ask yourself, can this be changed? The serenity prayer – God give me the courage to change what I can, to accept what I can't, and the wisdom to know the difference - is key to keeping sane, and to ensuring our eating behaviours don't go through the ceiling.

Caution:
In Mary's case, it became clear that she was ready to bring in a new focus. If however, your feeling about a "life unlived" is with regards some form of bereavement or life transition, this takes time and cannot simply be "filled in". It needs acknowledging, it takes its own time and has its own process. Attempting to bury any kind of bereavement tends to have an adverse effect, and hangs around to haunt you when you least suspect. If you are an emotional eater, you could find your eating behaviour escalating for no apparent reason.

The opposite is also true.

Collecting the evidence:
*Please make a **long** list and keep it somewhere you can keep adding to it!*

Your strengths:

-

-

-

-

-

What's GREAT about you? What do you appreciate about yourself?
What do others say they like about you?

-

-

-

-

-

-

I have only briefly dipped into the effects of core beliefs on our eating which could be a book in itself, but hopefully these few examples give enough insight to encourage further inquiry! I have listed below further reading and online links which go much more deeply into what is not only a fascinating subject, but provide the kind of self awareness that may help lessen any eating reactions tied to negative self belief.

For now though, let's look at some of those childhood "messages" that are still rattling the cage.

MESSAGES FROM THE PAST
and parental teaching…

I referred earlier to some of our beliefs being "swallowed whole" without our even realising and this constitutes much of what we would consider our value system: as we mature, this may shift from what we were taught as children, but it's surprising what sticks:

Waste not want not…
Clean up your plate…
It's a sin to leave food. The starving children of Africa etc etc…

Many of the directly food related messages have their place: there may have been good reason for these statements, especially if the food on the table is perhaps the hard earned produce of a meagre income.

Many of our parents, grandparents and great grandparents remember war time and post war rationing, which for some, brought levels of starvation that most of us, thank heaven, cannot nowadays remotely imagine so near to home.

Equally, understanding that what we are given is a privilege compared to the poor and needy teaches us to not take good fortune for granted. Early programming misfires though when our aversion to waste means we can't ever leave anything, and we're using ourselves as dustbins. A better lesson might be that of taking only what we need in the first place. Or allowing small children to take their own portion and learn accordingly, rather than dishing out portions on their behalf and expecting the lot to be eaten.

In contrast **"It's polite to leave a little food on the plate"** is about etiquette and status – designed not merely to show we have good grace and the quality of restraint, but further implying we can afford to do so!

Thankfully less in evidence these days, but perhaps a worthwhile up to date revision to help hold ourselves back might be about "leaving it in the shop", rather than the plate. *"Don't buy the bogofs!"* (Buy One Get One Free..)

And of the more fire and brimstone variety:

The meek shall inherit the earth, or we are all sinners.

Nothing like a good dose of guilt to exacerbate those eating behaviours, but the issue here is when part of our **unconscious** value system is at odds with how we live our lives and how we feel about ourselves.

How we believe we **ought** to be living, what we believe we **should or shouldn't** be doing, can create anything from a low level chronic distress to an overriding self negation. Life throws enough "curved balls" without the need for additional complication. If you're an emotional eater, sorting the wheat from the chaff, i.e. a genuinely challenging scenario, from what doesn't actually hold true, is always going to be helpful.

Messages and family expectation:
Many of these beliefs will come couched as expectations from the family: expectations not only of behaviour but also to do with achievement, expectations of caring for extended family, expectation of religious adherence etc.

One of my clients, a young second generation Hindu woman in her early twenties, abided lovingly to codes of conduct which included staying in the family home until such a time as she might marry.

Ever the dutiful daughter, her longing to go to a university in another part of the country was at odds with the expectation to stay home and cook and care for near and extended family.

Even though her loyalty was as exemplary as her behaviour, her desire to please her parents whom she loved deeply, clashed with her need to live an independent life, which ultimately she did. As a result she *felt* like a bad daughter, despite knowing this was not the case. Irrespective of her own views, she herself bought, in part, into the family belief system, so that her own internalised moral values were in conflict. Her work in progress, as it were, was to reconcile the contradictions and find peace within herself. Her eating was a powerful reaction to her distress and her weight visibly escalated whenever she returned home.

Can you think of any values you have which do not really serve you?

-

-

-

-

When do you feel guilty for something you know doesn't really hold ground, but you still feel guilty?

-

-

Similarly when do you feel irrationally disappointed with yourself?

-

-

Where and when do you find yourself compromised because of an outdated belief, or something you were taught as a child?

-

-

How often do the words "should/n't and ought/n't" echo somewhere in your mental conversation....?

-

-

How much is the issue with regards to an outside source of expectation, and how much have you bought into it yourself?

-

-

Where does your need to conform go against other needs?

-

-

Where does your need to please, go against your own needs?

-

-

-

Feeling you ought to be something, which goes against the grain of your nature, will always be a clue.

FAKE ETIQUETTE and PATTERNS of POLITENESS and the need to conform or please...

Carrying on from the above, **fake etiquette** is how I refer to subscribing to patterns of "polite behaviour" when they are as unnecessary as they are ill serving:

Many overeaters have a hard enough time without the "belief" that in order to be a good mother, a good host/ess, a good guest etc, there has to be food on offer all of the time or you that you have to eat whatever is offered, all of the time.

The "belief" that "If I do not offer enough I will not be good enough" or... "If I do not eat what has been bought (especially for celebration) I will be seen as rejecting the love that went into making it or buying it... *has no place* prioritizing itself over your need to be *healthy*, but that is exactly what is happening.

It may be that you hadn't realised what you were doing, hadn't thought of it that way. Which means you know now!

If though you feel bad about disappointing another person, or if you feel awkward about how you can say "thank you, but no thank you", there are ways of doing this that might be less threatening, which I expand on in the "Managing Situations and How to Say "No!" chapter, later on.

I am not suggesting that one is permanently boring or party pooper of the year. What I *am* suggesting, is that especially if you have weight related health issues, you really start to get clear on the exchange you are making.

I have lost count of the number of times a person allegedly desperate to reduce their weight, has sheepishly said they didn't like to disappoint everyone else at a celebration in their honour.

The underlying "belief system" goes like this:

If I don't do x y z (eat the cake / drink a glass / do whatever I believe is expected...) *then... they will think* less of me / not like me / think I'm boring / think I'm up on myself etc etc...

We all get caught once in a while, but it's *if* you're buying into this with such frequency that efforts to eat differently are continually thwarted, then you may choose to examine those beliefs! You also need to be clear as to whether the "excuse" is a cover for simply succumbing to temptation, and nothing to do with being polite. It really is very different. The approach is very different.

One is about feeling socially compromised, whether or not it is the case, and the belief that if you don't act in a particular way, there will be a cost, or a loss. There is often an **"if... then"** dialogue somewhere in the background of your mental conversation. The other, temptation, is about compromising one*self*!

I will often suggest strategy as a place to start, but if you find yourself stuck between oughts and shoulds, you may find it helpful to ask yourself whether it is **true.**

Is it **true** that I will be thought of in a different way... if I don't do what is expected?
If it is true, what will that **mean?**
Does it actually **matter?**
How often am I compromising my eating plans by conforming?
Is it contributing to my going astray more times than not?
If I were not worried about what people might think, not worried about the outcome, what would I **choose** to do?

Some years back a lady called Wanda used to have regular business trips to Japan. Over and above the effect of jet lag on her hunger, she felt her dining and entertainment "schedule" was making it near impossible to keep to any kind of moderate eating regime, and that refusal would be taken badly. Her need to find a way through became urgent, as her increasing weight on long haul journeys was exacerbating circulatory problems and risk of deep vein thrombosis.

Unpacking this, there were several assumptions jangling around Wanda's bag of beliefs:
The first – was the felt necessity to eat a lot, or eat everything.
Was this true?

Culturally, this was not actually the case. Providing she ate some, this would be acceptable.

Second – (since there were a number of dining events on any day...) was the belief that if she chose not to eat, it would make the business client feel awkward eating alone, and put focus on her dieting, instead of the client. This in turn would have an effect on continued commercial relations, which might mean she'd lose the client or the campaign. Ultimately, if she lost enough campaigns, she'd lose her job, and if she lost her job, she'd be unable to pay her mortgage and lose her home. Wow!! No small chain reaction here!

What was true, and what wasn't?

It was true that the client needed to feel included, and relaxed.

It was true that the focus needed to be on the client.

It was true that a happy client is a lot more conducive to further business relations than one who feels awkward.

Was there a way around it?

What Wanda realised was that if she had some reason for dietary restriction which could be made clear prior to her arrival, the Japanese would most likely be more than keen as "good hosts" to accommodate those needs. This would be deemed seemly as well as culturally correct and then would not become an issue after the fact.

Her plan for the next trip, which for the record worked well, was to create more coffee meetings than actual dining events, and to stipulate her preference for fish and protein and her need to avoid wheat and sugar.

What this story flags up is the power of assumption: until we picked it apart, Wanda's leap from "not conforming" to losing her job and home had not been fully recognised, but was having a concerning knock on effect on her weight and health.

How much of your overeating is due to a sense of obligation or fear of a particular consequence?

-

-

How much of your assumption is true?

-

-

If it is true, do you have options, can you approach it differently?

-

-

As ever:

What do you want?

What do you choose to do?

What are you willing to do?

What are you able to do?

DISTORTED THINKING...
"I've Blown it!" and other things we tell ourselves...

How often have you begun a diet or a more sensible eating regime only to feel you've blown it at some point or other?

What usually happens after?

Do you brush yourself off and resume the previous good work? Or do you comfort or punish yourself for the transgression by eating twice as much?

The problem here is that over and above whatever situation has taken you off track, the "I've blown it" factor is the bit that really does the damage.

As you fill in your Eating Behaviour Blueprint in increasing detail, you will start to notice whatever combination of social, emotional and physical gets in the way and trips you up. However many times you fall down a hole, at some point all hindsight becomes foresight and one day you will find yourself averting that hole.

"I've blown it" type of thinking though, *is* one of the holes.

It is a kind of knee jerk, black and white thinking reaction which leaps from one extreme to another allowing no middle ground for repair. We're either 100% right or 100% wrong, a total success or a total failure. It's an All or Nothing reaction which in eating terms makes it one of *the* most fattening thought processes as well as one of the hallmarks of yo yo dieting, so it is really worth catching in action!

Variations on the *All or Nothing* theme show the same *either / or* polarisation:

I'm on a diet	*or*	*I'm off the diet*
I'm in control	*or*	*I'm out of control*
I'm perfect	*or*	*I'm rubbish*
I'm a success	*or*	*I'm a failure*
I'm good	*or*	*I'm bad*
It's all going well	*or*	*Everything's ruined!*

… translates as….

If I can't get it right, I'll give up   *or*   *I was doing so well but now I've ruined everything*

…and so on.

What this type of thinking says is that there is no room for the kind of mistakes which are part and parcel of learning. Instead of taking note of what happened, (the purpose of the spectrums and your Eating Behaviour Blueprint), the modus operandi is often a slightly crazed eating reaction.

Whilst frustration or upset or disappointment is completely understandable, acting it out over and again by eating even more does not serve your aim. What it's effectively doing is bouncing off one wall and hitting another. For any Trekkies out there, imagine Spock's quizzical response to this strange behaviour! As I state in my introduction, most people are focussed on what they are eating, but once you catch this reaction and put your foot in the door as it were, you really will be on the road to success.

Do any of these reactions sound like you?

When, where, or with whom do you noticing it happening most often?

Once you spot these in action, take note of what happens to your eating in the time that follows, and how long it takes you to get back on track.

Your work, initially, is to find whatever means you have of bringing the usual reaction to a halt, and going back to where you were. The impulse to dump what you'd begun so well may be overwhelming, but that is *only* because it's what you've got used to doing, it's been your normal behaviour for so long. It's the kind of conditioned reflex I described in the chapter on Habits so it may take time to instil a new response.

Even if you don't succeed for a while, don't be tempted to act out a parallel process with your efforts and ditch even trying the moment there's a glitch!

However unfamiliar it seems, try to use a different way of saying things to yourself or more balanced language to produce a different outcome.

Balanced language...

Saying to yourself, "I'd *prefer* to have been perfect but what I have done is ok", or "I may not be completely successful but I'll get there", or "Every day in every way I'm getting past this glitch!" may sound like the understatements of the century but say it to yourself anyway. It will hit the right button at some point.

Make up your own positive statements, or affirmations. When you find yourself laughing in the process, it's already lessened the negative feeling that usually tips you over, so you're onto a winner!

Again, should you feel quaintly ridiculous muttering apparent platitudes to yourself, take yourself lightly and remember humour is far more effective than shame.

If you *are* a perfectionist, and you cannot see past this, then think of it this way:

"**Perfection**" in dieting terms *is* being able to hold the *balance* between your impulses and your thoughts as much as your food.

Otherwise the food keeps following the impulse!

"Perfection"... *is* finding a way to prevent the extreme reaction back to overeating so you can hold a ***balance*** in the middle, *enough* of the time.

This may take time as it's as compelling as it's automatic but you really will get there!!

Catch the reaction in action....!

In her book "Confidence Works..."[53] Glenda McMahon describes different types of self defeating, negative thinking styles which in one way or other are all "holes in the road". They frequently precipitate bad eating habits and get us absolutely nowhere except back to where we began. Recognising them and noticing where they keep cropping up is essential, both to understanding what on earth is going on all the time, i.e. regaining a truer perspective, and so moderating the eating and maintaining a better relationship with food. See if any of these relate to you, including the All or Nothing above, and notice if and when they occur before an eating reaction.

Don't worry if initially you feel unable to stop the reflex from your thought to your overeating. Simply catching the reaction in action is a great start! Remember your detective! Observe, write it down, collect the evidence! The more you can expand your list of "I can't believe I *do* that!!", the more successfully you will get your foot in the door, sooner rather than later!

Catastrophising:
Exaggerating the impact of events and convincing yourself that if something goes wrong it will be a disaster and you won't be able to cope. For example:

"If I get a craving it will be unbearable."
"If I lapse on this diet everything will be ruined."
"If I make a mistake I will lose my job. "

---

[53] Confidence Works - Learn to be Your Own Life Coach by Gladeana McMahon SPCK Publishing 2001.

It's like an extreme version of "I've blown it" but it often kicks into action before any mistake has even been made. There's an assumption of failure or "catastrophe" before you even start.

Jumping to negative conclusions:
Drawing a negative conclusion when there is no evidence to support it. A form of **mind reading**, you might decide someone is reacting negatively toward you and react on that basis, (eg comfort eating) without checking it out. For example:

"That person is yawning / looking elsewhere / has interrupted me twice…. So I must be boring to listen to…"

Fortune telling and predicting the future:
You anticipate what will happen without evidence to support it. You're convinced your prediction is an already established fact and react on that basis. Worse, negative expectation is often self fulfilling. For example:

"S/he hasn't called yet so I know they're not interested… "
"I'm going to fail, so why begin…?"
"I'll never be able to change… my eating habits / drinking" etc...

Mistaking feelings for facts:
Confusing facts for feelings or beliefs. For example:

"I feel a failure, so I must be a failure".
No matter how strong a feeling is, it doesn't make it a fact.

Discounting the positive:
Rejecting or trivialising achievements and positive experiences by insisting they "don't count" or for some reason were "just lucky". For example:

"She only gave me that compliment because she knows how bad I am feeling…" or "I only did well because there wasn't much competition… "

Interestingly where this happens with great frequency, is when we are given compliments. There is a curious "pattern of politeness" that somehow acts as though it is improper to accept the "gift". Actually by implication we reject the compliment and negate the act of "giving".

Mental filtering:
Similar to the above but you see only the negative and dwell on them so much it distorts your view of a person or situation.

It might be about your own accomplishments where one constructive or more negative comment offsets a 100 good ones, or it might be a pretext for extending a grudge! For example:

"I'll never forget they let me down that time."

Generalisation:
Assuming that because something has gone wrong, it will always do so. We draw conclusions from a one off event. For example:

"I always lapse. I'll never be able to stop overeating." Or..
"Fat people don't get promoted..."

Generalisation and extreme words:
Extreme statements are only rarely true.

Always: You always leave me to sort things out. I always have to clear up after you.

Never: I can never do what I really want to do. I'll never get anything right. You never listen to anything I say.

Nobody / Everyone / They: Nobody ever notices how hard I try. Everyone else is better than me. They say what comes round goes around.

Personalisation and blame:

Blaming ourselves...
Assuming when bad things happen it is always your fault. Taking too much responsibility for other people's feelings and behaviour when it neither stems from you nor is about you. For example:

"So and so is in a really bad mood. It must be something I've said or done..."

Blaming others and Excuse Making:
In contrast to the above we take no responsibility and blame other people and situations.

"It's not fair!" is the excuse making variety of blame whereby comparison with others serves little save to foster resentment.

Often based on a false perception about others and the world around us, the "why me?" or "no-one else has this problem" victim stance keeps a person safe from being fully accountable.

Taking things personally:
Feeling easily criticized, disliked or rejected when it isn't necessarily the case. For example:

"S/he didn't ask my opinion because s/he doesn't value me."

Self put downs:
This involves putting yourself down or undervaluing yourself. It is often an extreme reaction to a situation where we feel we've made an error or not done well enough. For example:

"I'm completely useless."
"I'm weak / stupid / ugly..."
"I don't deserve any better.."

Should statements and pressuring words:
"Shoulds", "oughts" and "musts" are often used when people want to try

to motivate themselves to do better or try harder, but instead they tend to make people feel pressured and resentful so motivation actually decreases.

Should: I should have done better. You should have let me know.
Must: I must get this right. I must not make a mistake.
Have to: I have to get there on time. I have to make this relationship work.
Ought to: I ought never lose my temper. I ought to get there on time.

All of the above are common enough thinking distortions but what needs spotting is if they lead to overeating more often than not.

- Your first step is always simply to **notice** you are doing this.
  By noticing, there is already a **separation** between the thought and the usual follow up, such as the overeating. By noticing, you are catching it midstream and already putting your foot in the door, preventing the distortion from hitting its target!

- As always, use your "policeperson's notebook"... and **write it down!**
  Or put it in your phone, whatever, but you are far more likely to effect a change by doing this. Some part of you will think "Ye gads! I'm actually serious!".

- If you're not sure, **ask a friend** or someone you value whether you tend to react in a particular way, or jump to conclusions etc.

  You might find their observation enlightening:
  Some years ago after I'd used a "jush-ing" sound to describe something, my brother began laughing and said "Do you know you do that about ten times a day?". It wasn't that serious, but I replied indignantly that I did no such thing and he was being ridiculous. "Suit yourself" he replied, laughing even more, "now I've told you you'll start noticing!".
  Ten times a day?! He'd underestimated its frequency! I was horrified! But it's an eye opener as to just how much we do without realising!

- Ask yourself, **is it true?** Is it true some of the time or all of the time?

296

- *Check it out.* What is the evidence for whatever you believe? If it exists, as above, is it the case all of the time or just some of the time?

- *Check out the pay offs.* Do you benefit from the thinking distortion? For example, if the slightest thing makes you believe you'll fail, or you feel there's "no point" to something, does it in fact give you a get out clause, an escape clause? You might feel like it's letting you off the hook, but your eating behaviour and your weight will indicate otherwise.

- *Check out the link with your eating behaviours.* If your thinking distortions upset you a lot of the time, and you're an emotional eater, it's going to add impetus to the need to review!

Notice the situation. What are your thoughts? Your main feeling? Your (eating) behaviour?

For instance:
Situation: Someone might have angered you at work but you don't say anything.
Negative Thinking: You make an assumption they don't value you.
Feeling: You feel upset as well as angry.
Behaviour: You end up eating a packet of biscuits left out on the desk.

You might also find that it rarely stops there. The cycle continues. For example:
Feeling: Now you are even more upset as you have eaten so much.
Negative thinking: "I've blown it. No point being sensible now...." etc.
Eating behaviour: Buys pizza / cake / etc on way home.

and so on... So...

Think of your own example. Write down the process, and *do* write this, as truly it makes a difference. Now start to ask yourself what might be a healthier response?

How might you see things differently? How might you *behave* differently?

What might you do instead?

Remember again, we're not building Rome in a day. If you expect insight to immediately be followed by a corrective action, you may succeed, but you may also be disappointed and we're back to the critical, castigating "parent"! Habits have a nice tight hold, and the ones with a benefits package attached, whether giving into temptation or alleviating an emotion or discomfort, may not comply straight away with your desire for their immediate removal. If only!

Even if each time you are able to look back and realise what happened, to see the tippet-toe stepping stones to the giant hole and know what you would *prefer* to do differently in future, (note balanced, *not* All or None use of language!) that is a *giant* leap forward!

Finally...

Practise saying "Thank You!" when you receive a compliment. Do not justify or negate! It's far more gratifying for the person giving the compliment, (ye gads, they just accepted my gift!) and it works wonders for your wellbeing!

At some point, all hindsight becomes foresight. All mistakes become grist for the mill. It's all information!

DISTORTED THINKING…
"I'll Just Have One!" and other porky pies[54]…

Alert! Child at Large!

Many years ago my mother and I were breakfasting on the outside terrace of the rather wonderful Victoria Falls Hotel in Zimbabwe. Engrossed as we were in conversation, we barely noticed the paw attaching itself to our pile of croissants till its owner, a young monkey, glanced upward with wide eyed alarm as we caught him in the act. Frozen to the spot but not deterred, he covered his eyes with his remaining paw as he fed himself our croissants with the other. Neither was he to be rushed. Keeping his eyes covered, he continued chewing till all was gone, casting one last slightly guilty look in our direction as he skulked back into the bushes.

Impressed as I remain at his method, it brings to mind the many things we do, not only to "hide from sight" but to hide from ourselves. With child like ingenuity, we somehow convince ourselves that "if we can't see it, it can't be there," or variations of… and rarely is this more apparent than with the fabrications we concoct to treat ourselves or to let ourselves off the hook.

See if you recognise *any* of these…

- I'll only have one

- Just this once / on this occasion…

- It needs finishing / it's only a small bit…

- In for a penny in for a pound…

- I've been so good …I deserve…

- I'm so tired / upset / I deserve

- It's been a long day, I've worked so hard… I deserve…

- It doesn't count unless I'm at the table

- It doesn't count on the run / in the car / on the train…

---

[54] Porky pies: Cockney rhyme for fibs and lies.

- I always have a salad to start (so the rest doesn't count...)
- I'll start tomorrow / next Monday / next lifetime ...

Add your own favourites...!!

-

-

-

-

-

-

Endearing as it is, we give ourselves permission on the pretext that it's only temporary, and somehow continue to keep kidding ourselves over the years and despite evidence to the contrary.

We are so good at this and so sophisticated at finding ways around that normally sane part of ourselves, that we have not so much patterns of politeness as patterns of collusion, so that when offered some delicacy we can feign restraint then act as though obliged: another's prompting of "Go on, go on, go on," and "no, I mustn't, really shouldn't..." (if not our own internal conversation!) invariably followed by a mopping of the brow and "Oh, if you absolutely insist, alright then..." pretence of giving in for the sake of decorum!

There is something incurably compelling about indulging a naughty child but it is exactly that "child within" whose perverse reasoning power needs reckoning with if we are not forever to be tempted astray!

The "oh well, life's short / life is for living / you only live once..." rationale has tremendous appeal and were it not for the outcome, indeed, why would it matter?

The answer is it wouldn't, and moreover there is something about being mischievous, giving ourselves a little treat and letting ourselves off here and there that is as heart warming as it is playful. We also **need** to let go once in a while. It is **only** when the indulgences add up and we're losing control that we play at our peril.

One lady in her fifties had told me her downfall over the months were the jelly tots she kept "for her son" which she'd then end up eating every week or so. Assuming she'd been a late mum to have such a young child, I finally let go of discretion and asked his age. Thirty five. Yes, thirty five. He must really have missed those jelly tots!

A variation on the "I'll only have one" but starting at the point of purchase is when we delude ourselves we are "saving" on discounted offers:

REALITY CHECK the FALSE ECONOMIES...

No "economy buying" if history proves otherwise! If what you buy for the week gets eaten in far less than a week, regularly, simply because it is *there... STOP!*

It may take a while to fully realise that you are rarely ever "sensible *this* time," but at some point down the line you may really have to trust ... that you simply can't be trusted!! That, however, is the beginning of *real* trust and taking note of how you operate!

If you are an inveterate over shopper, then while shopping on line might seem more expensive, delivery charge tagged on etc, you might want to do the maths as they say, and check whether this is actually true. Providing you are *not* hungry when purchasing online and hence likely to the same antics as when you are wandering Pinocchio like down the food aisles, you may well find that you're buying for need rather than for whim benefits your purse as well as your body!

Make a list of your favourite excuses and the pretexts that go with them. Ask yourself whether it is true, or a dirty rotten lie:

More of your favourite excuses:

-

-

-

-

-

Ask yourself:

*How **often** do I say this?*

*Is it **true?** i.e. do I really have only one, start the next day etc etc?*

Do I often regret it later?

What is the main feeling later on, i.e. upset, regret, anger, guilt, disappointment...?

How much does this disrupt my eating plan?

Is it contributing toward my weight gain?

Ask yourself:

Will I be pleased with my choice in 2 hours time?

Word to the wise:
What you do **not** want to do is to berate or get angry with the part of you that keeps doing this. It tends to be counterproductive and more usually has the effect of a controlling parent on a wayward child and ends up with a tantrum. Instead of compliance you can find yourself rebelling, ***even when the conversation is in your own head:***

The self reproaching part of you that is disappointed with whatever you've been doing and castigates *is* like a criticising parent, while the child like part says "See if I care!" which translates behaviourally to two fingers in the air and carrying on regardless... If you are able to exert discipline to good effect, this is of course more than fine. It is when a negative reaction is having an adverse effect, over and again, that castigation is futile and we need a different approach.

Eric Berne, founder of Transactional Analysis, describes beautifully how the internalized "ego states" of Child and Parent operate upon each other, to our detriment or benefit[55]. Thankfully, the presence of an Adult ego state is the one which while discerning, is accepting, non judgemental,

---

[55] Eric Berne's Games People Play 1964 describes The Ego State (or Parent-Adult-Child) model www.ericberne.com/transactional-analysis

and takes on board all relevant information, in other words, as full a picture as possible.

If you can, act with yourself as you would with a child.

Take their hand and as lovingly as possible lead them to a more engaging distraction. This is where your list of distractions, (that over time you will know to have handy..!) comes into play. Literally.

Just to remind yourself, make yet another list here of whatever would most quickly grab your attention elsewhere whenever you most need.

Have *fun* with it though!

DISTRACTIONS LIST: things to do, places to go, people to call... aka "things to take mind away from impulse" list:

-

-

-

-

-

Sometimes trusting that you can't be trusted, in one or two matters, is your safest route forward!

PART 5:
TRICKS OF THE TRADE

MANAGING SITUATIONS AND HOW TO SAY "NO"

One of the advantages of being with fellow weight watchers is hearing situations which put you one step ahead: there are so many times we get caught short, or realise after the fact, that a different response would have got us off the hook, or taken the focus away from our trying to abstain! It's challenging enough overcoming our own temptation, the voice in our own head that eggs us on, without adding other people into the equation.

I have my own examples but was so impressed by Erin Whitehead's online blog, "Ways to Say No to Food Pushers"[56] that I recommend having a look: she refers to situations in which a temptation arises as The Push, followed by an alternative response.

Although saying "no" might be in response to an invitation to eat, it can be *any* situation where giving in or relenting ends *up* with overeating as a *reaction.*

It's that chain reaction once again, between situation and behaviour, you need to look out for.

Golden rule... sound like you mean it!
Do take stock however that if you say "no", you need to look and sound like you mean it! If our tone or posture or expression looks like we're half hearted turning something down, we're giving a double message and people are quick to pick up on ambivalence. Patterns of collusion then pop up and we're into the "Go on, go on, go on" goon show!

Golden rule... prepare before you go...
Because temptation already puts us on the back foot, it really is a good idea to always go through any social situation in your mind *before* you get there. "Seeing how it goes" is either a recipe for disaster or a get out clause with an intent to see whether your urge to indulge will win out over your

---

[56] Erin Whitehead: Nice Ways to say "No" to Food Pushers
http://www.sparkpeople.com/resource/nutrition

need to be careful. You can guess which usually wins! Is it for example, a seated event, is it a buffet, might you be able to mingle with something small on your plate so people don't constantly add to temptation by offering more and commenting if you abstain?

Consider ahead as well, who will be there. Is there anyone whose company irritates you or makes you feel ill at ease in any way, aggravating an emotional need to overeat, if not then, then later? Remember this can just as easily be family, or a partner's family, which might be all the more tricky if it is a regular event. It is not unusual for people to feel at once focussed upon because of their weight, whilst expected to satisfy the host with greater than usual indulgence.

Working out strategies in advance, even by virtue of bolstering your ability to hold your ground, or engaging the support of someone reliable, might be an essential part of your "practise"!

Equally, if you're planning on a level of restraint, do *not* go starving! Have something small before you go!

This isn't about having to permanently abstain: it's about getting on with a settled decision so that losing weight, if that's your aim, doesn't take forever. Or if your aim is to stay stable, then knowing ahead which occasions are liable to take you off track will increase your skill at weight holding.

Along with having become much more familiar with where your social commitments and general lifestyle put you at risk, the Rolling Event Calendar at the end of this chapter will help you see at a glance where you are with this.

Head space and time to think on your feet...
There will always be a moment when we're caught short, suddenly asked to join someone for a bite etc, and lack of time to think of a stalling tactic is most often when we end up, in a nanosecond, abdicating our best laid plans. Again, this is not about leading a life devoid of spontaneity and fun: it's about having enough boundaries so we **can** have fun when we choose and not "waste calories".

This said, if you've made your mind up on any given day that you'll be sticking to a particular eating regime, that settled decision ahead of time makes everything *so* much easier.

Each morning, check: What is my intention today? What might sabotage that intention? Is there a way around it?

If caught short:

Ask yourself:
Am I actually hungry? and **Will this be socially or emotionally valuable?** to decide whether you genuinely want or need to eat.

If an off the cuff, face to face invitation finds you stuck for an answer, get yourself some thinking time by saying you need to excuse yourself for a minute, like popping to the bathroom, or having to make a quick call, during which time you can devise your get out tactic! Sad, I know, but needs must! Looking and sounding flustered as you search for a way out appears odd at the least and at worst can seem rude.

Problems with portion control and desperate measures!
Looking like you're trying to watch your weight can attract unwanted attention at the best of times but be particularly inappropriate professionally.

Some years ago a lady who'd been slimming for her wedding day suddenly found herself roped into a work conference "banquet" the week before her final dress fitting. Frantic with concern, as she found portion control under such circumstances almost impossible, she decided to use the "jippy tummy" excuse.

The bonus with this, which lest it start attracting concern about your health should **only** be used as a last resort, is that while feigning huge disappointment and thus satisfying hosts or peers that every ounce of you would have wished otherwise, you know you'll be left in peace: no-one **ever** wants to think bowel motions at the dinner table, so it's very taboo-ness ensures success and also protects you from yourself!

Feel bad saying no?

Many people find it very difficult to say "no" and somehow feel obligated. Yet being unable to say *no* often results in feeling resentful as well as over extended, and that can again lead to emotional overeating.

When we cannot say *no*, it means we are equally unable to set limits and boundaries or make clear our needs so it may *seem* (distorted thinking) as if others use us, or take advantage, and "get their own way".

This may be true, but it may also be that in the absence of reading our minds or knowing us better, they have gone ahead with what suits them, and indeed what they might believe suits you, if no other discussion took place.

Having a few phrases to hand, already "prepared", can be a real life saver!

Can you think of different ways to say "No thank you" such as "If you don't mind I won't for the moment" etc.?

Make a list:

-

-

-

-

Make a list also, of reasons you would find acceptable to give for refusal, such as "Thank you I've just eaten" or "I have a phone call to make but thanks, another time" etc.

-

-

-

-

Make a list of reasons to refuse a particular item:

For example: "Thanks, I'm not drinking tonight as I'm driving" or "Thanks, I'm off wheat / sugar / at the moment – doctor's orders", which is now much more widely accepted. (Perhaps caution with the doctor's orders lest it elicits more of the wrong kind of attention!), or one of Erin's: "Thanks, I just had some... it was delicious". Even if they suspect otherwise at least it you are paying a compliment so you shouldn't get pinned to the wall!

-

-

-

-

-

-

Follow up and ensure the subject is forgotten by moving the focus elsewhere:

Make a list of questions or comments to change the subject with speed at a social gathering when food is offered, or if the question of your not eating something looks like it's about to get too much attention. Additionally if your eating escalates in situations which make you socially nervous, having some questions to hand to elicit conversation from others can be remarkably helpful, as well as shifting focus with grace:

"How are you / your children / pet dog / parrot / etc etc doing at the moment?" or "How are you finding ...?" xyz topical subject... usually engages attention elsewhere with ease, and again does the trick while being socially well regarded.

The more you become adept at this, the easier it gets to stick to your intent!

-

-

-

-

Returning to polite refusal however -

Do you find the thought of saying no, however well put, easy or challenging?

-

Ask yourself:

How do you feel when someone else says "no" to you?

-

-

What is your belief about someone who is able to do this?

-

-

List at least two situations in which you would like to have said "no" when someone asked for a favour you weren't happy about.

-

-

-

List two or more occasions when you would like to have said "no" to something food related.

-

-

-

Complete the sentence below about what you believe might happen when you say "no". (i.e. "If I say no....I won't be liked, I'll sound like my mother" etc...).

When I say "no"...

-

-

-

Can you think of times this would not be true?

-

-

Ask yourself:

What is it you fear?

-

-

Who do you most fear saying "no" to and why?

-

-

-

Who do you feel you can most easily say "no" to, or in what situation are you more able to say "no"?

-

-

What is the difference?

-

-

Can you think of anyone you know who is able to say "no" with such grace and tact it's hardly an issue?

-

-

Might you feel able to follow their example?

-

-

List two situations you believe you could say "no" to within a month. They need not be directly food related. It might not be a direct "no", but there will be a definite boundary.

-

-

"No" as an answer *may* put out or upset the other person, especially if they are accustomed to your saying "yes" and have possibly even banked on it. In fact if it's been going on for years, it could be an implicit part of the relationship and you may initially get the very kind of response you most fear! This is why when you first experiment with "no", (or, "no if you don't mind, I'm not able..." which is a little less dogmatic!) start with tiny things that won't make *such* a difference to the other person, although this isn't about them, it's to make it easier for you!

Start with small steps: No need to put your head in the lion's mouth *just* yet as it would only frighten you back into compliance! Get confidence initially with small refusals, or drawing a line which won't rock the boat too much!

As I mentioned before people are quick to pick up on ambivalence so unless you sound like you mean it, you may find yourself pushed at first. But keep practising.

Often it may not even be about someone trying to get you to *do* something but simply turning down an invitation.

Their response is not your responsibility...

A person's reaction to our setting a boundary does not mean we have to renege on our resolve if we genuinely need to hold our ground. Discomfort, pain or upset does not mean it is wrong to say "no", though tears or reproach are often unconscious "survival" techniques to make sure needs gets met, and if we let it, becomes emotional blackmail. Taking a leap from Eleanor Roosevelt's claim, that no one can make you feel inferior without your consent... it takes two and if something is happening repeatedly, (see Games People Play[57]) you are as much party to the interaction as are they. Responding differently can feel uncomfortable, and more so when we take responsibility, or feel to blame for the outcome. Assuming however you have not been abducted by pirates or are in some kind of hijack situation, we deceive ourselves when we protest "I had to..., they made me" etc and besides, there is *always* a time when we are more than able to hold our ground, when we choose, even if it isn't with regard to food or drink.

---

[57] Games People Play 1964 Eric Berne.

What you'll find though is that as your voice has more certainty, people take you more seriously and there'll be less of a problem.

Ask yourself:

When, with whom and in what situations have I held my ground with relative ease?

-

-

-

-

Why should this be different?

-

-

-

Do I feel exposed, or vulnerable in some way? Do I have the feeling that people guess I have problems with overeating? If so, is this true, and what if it is?

-

-

-

-

Sometimes the ***felt*** sense can be overpowering: one of my group who was otherwise more than able to hold her own in many ways would never ask for a mug of hot water in her local cafe, even when her friends were all getting hot drinks, so she could easily have got away with doing this. Her overwhelming sense was that, rationally or not, "everyone (else in the cafe) would know I was on a diet", which would then lead to judgements that she "shouldn't have put on so much weight in the first place".

If you realise you feel like this in some situations, it is *possible* that recognition alone may enable you to click your fingers and release the reaction, but it is equally likely that you may freeze on the spot when caught in the same scenario.

Again, simply notice what is happening. Where in your body are you feeling the strength of the emotion? Are your cheeks hot and flushed with embarrassment? Has your breathing almost stopped as if it will lessen your being noticed? See if you are able to catch yourself in the moment and let go, or at least tell yourself it really is ok, however much you may feel disinclined to believe it at first. Then check the evidence. Ask yourself whether it is true that everyone will be making judgements, or that they will know you are on a diet etc. The late Martha Graham, (American dancer and choreographer) used to say that what other people think of us is really none of our business. Not always easy to abide by, but a good one to aim for perhaps!

Eventually you will loosen the strength of the emotion, but it can take time, and patience takes us back to the loving parent, or Adult ego state of the last chapter.

Write down any situations where the emotional reaction, or felt sense seems to fix you to the spot. Where you feel emotionally trapped and unable to act differently?

-

-

-

What do you fear people might be thinking?

-

-

If they were thinking whatever it is you fear, what would that mean?

-

-

Is it any of their business?

-

Does it reflect more accurately your own judgement about yourself?

-

What might you prefer to say or do?

-

-

Make saying "yes" a genuine choice...

Being able to set limits when you need gives you choice but make sure saying "yes" when you do, is genuine and not quietly eroding you and affecting your eating behaviours, and hence potentially your weight and health.

Powerful martyrs or victims are those who, unable or unwilling to state their case "suffer in silence" and often assert themselves in some other way to exact the compromise or result they desire.

Conversely being with someone who sets boundaries means we know where we stand. Who would you rather be with? How would you rather be?

Caution: Social eating... saying "no" to ourselves!

Try to resist bemoaning in public all the things you "dare not have" or "can't possibly have" on a menu. It seems to have the effect of throwing down the gauntlet, and even assuming this is to bolster your intent and not to deliberately attract attention to your amazing restraint, it can be misinterpreted and usually invokes a barrage of questions about why you feel the need. I used to do this without realising and couldn't understand why all the focus on my eating. Worse, if you do need to lose weight, an uninvited interrogation as to the nature of your diet, your health, and your likelihood of success or failure can be toe-curlingly unwelcome.

Avoid at all costs!

Special events:

Again using the Rolling Event Calendar at the end of this chapter, decide ahead of time what is important for you: finding yourself either ahead of or during events with an oscillating should I / shouldn't I argument going round and round your head, neither makes for a fun occasion nor allows you to be fully open to enjoy yourself, or others.

Of course your granny's 80th or your child's 21st are occasions you may well want to share. Who wouldn't? It is when there is one after the other after the other and it's a cake trail of non stop "reasons", that you might want to question what's important, and how much your health is an issue. It goes back to *what do you actually want?*

If it's your *own* birthday that's being celebrated and you know ahead of time people will be expecting you to indulge, again, whose birthday *is* it and are you happy to indulge your friends at the expense of your health or what is truly meaningful to you? What would those friends think if they knew you were sacrificing your goal just to keep them happy? We're back to a variation on saying "no" but it will be an awful lot easier way ahead of time to let people know that what you really want *is* a departure perhaps from the norm. Often as not it is more about tradition and feeling maybe like you are spoiling something very special for others. So if your choice, or need, *is* to stick to a regime, let them know how *important it is to you and how much it means.* Providing it is done sufficiently in advance, you won't then be "cheating" or depriving them of the enjoyment of giving.

If too the thought of addressing this is upsetting or difficult, at least ask yourself the questions posed earlier, i.e. What is it that I fear? If I do xyz what do I fear people will think of me? What do I believe might happen? What does this mean? What might be the worst outcome?

Sometimes to get to the bottom of an issue, to discover what is really ailing, you have to keep going with the "If....Then" question and answer process till the nugget at the bottom is revealed! Peeling away the layers, be it gently, is once again the detective in action!

The planned dinner party:
If it's a once a week event, it can be easy enough to fit in, (see my 4-2-1 budget / banquet later on) or to "pay it forward" ahead of time.

Sometimes though, when we decide to bite the bullet and seriously reduce our intake, (which could be a reduction to *normal* eating if you've been *over*eating...) then we could be waiting for ever if you try to bypass every invitation, and more so if you are fortunate in having a wide social circle.

If then you are going to be remotely obvious – you may want to consider calling whoever's cooking *ahead* of time. *Way* ahead of time. It is so the norm now for at least one of one's friends to have a "dietary difference", be it gluten free, nut free, vegetarian etc etc, that it is less likely to be mocked and moreover gives your host the chance to be amazingly gracious and come up with the goods. In contrast to this, my pet hate over the years (yes, it's a Room 101 hate for anyone familiar with that silly programme!) is the person who, "not wanting to make a fuss", does just that on arrival at the table. In one stroke they are a darn nuisance and have deprived me of my opportunity to shine as a wonderful hostess! And that could, by the way, be someone who would love to come but really might prefer to eat remarkably little. If they have checked ahead, their company is hopefully all that really matters, but, balking at etiquette as I do on occasion, it is none the less good form!

The restaurant:
Again as above, a lot may depend on whether this is a regular feature or the occasional outing.

If you are in charge, and especially if it's on the professional agenda, it is a great idea to amass a list of restaurants that work well for you: whilst as an inveterate overeater when it comes to portion control, I can bemoan the aesthetically scant offerings of say French cuisine at times, it is one big bonus when it comes to enforced restraint. In addition to which, being a regular at certain eateries means you can probably get away with requests before arrival. One place I went to knew never to serve me bread. I have to confess there was often a moment when I wished vehemently for the ritual to be ignored but I couldn't bear the indignity of having to explain my reversal of decision! Job done!

If conversely it's not up to you, your restaurant outing cannot be avoided and falls smack bang into your new eating regime / diet etc, take the initiative and check the menu ahead of time. Once again you will arrive with a relatively settled decision with far less chance of temptation getting the better of you in the heat of the moment. Besides which few people will take issue with you passing on dessert or whatever. (Do try though to keep your beady eyes off other people's scraping remains. It's vaguely off putting and gives the game away which to my shame, I know all too well!)

Finally if you are absolutely stuck you might consider the little white lie which allows you to turn up later in the meal, or for coffee. Again most of this is down to thinking ahead and a bit of ingenuity.

The pub:
Football season / rugby season...

The first time I gave up smoking, (yes, there were several attempts before lift off!) I had to stop going to the pub. A temptation too far was always the inexorable coupling of a drink and a cigarette so I avoided, for the duration, anywhere which could undermine my intent.

For many however, time at the pub has greater social meaning and might be less willingly dropped, and whilst legislation has put paid to the smoking, that still leaves the snacks and the alcohol: one of my clients, whose weight was now posing serious health risks, knew he didn't really have a choice, and was prepared to override his ritual nights out with the lads for a given time, but was fraught as to how he would manage the rugby season: no *way* would he miss the ritual, after the match gatherings, and no *way* could he see himself holding firm to his resolve, and sipping a lemon and lime!

Given we had two months till the season began, I asked whether he'd be willing to cross that hurdle when it arrived, on the basis that improved health might put him in a very different frame of mind, which he couldn't remotely imagine at the present time. That, as it turned out was exactly what happened: fast forward two stone lighter, lowered blood pressure and cholesterol, pain free joints and far more energy, Andy not only felt a hundred per cent better but was enjoying a renewed vigour, which no amount of ritualised drinking with the clan was going to jeopardise: he let some of the men know ahead of time so he'd have support, and whilst he did eventually bring alcohol back into the equation, it was heavily interspersed with pints of water!

The pointers here once again, are knowing which choices are *most important* to you; planning, where possible *ahead* of time so the rewards give strength to resolve, and working out at the very least, a compromise. In Andy's case informing a few of the guys avoided the pitfall of giving in simply to avoid being questioned, and moreover won respect as well as support.

The holiday:

If treating yourself, having a reward for all your hard work, is part and parcel of your weight gain, you might want to choose holidays with care: apart from being amongst others, family, friends, who probably won't delight in the ongoing diet at this time and may feel cheated, the opportunity for temptation along with the "it's my downtime" mindset can make saying "no" to *ourselves* a near nigh impossible challenge.

So unless for some reason it is set in stone, maybe don't go for that cruise, or for that matter the all inclusive, until you are more than adept at weight management: not only do we run into "I've paid for it so I'm darn well going to have it," value for money mindset, (even when what you've spent on dieting comprises far more...) but worse it presents temptation at every turn. Is it *really* a holiday if you are struggling from breakfast through to dinner to hold yourself back from the brink? Hardly! If you know you are going to really enjoy your food, choose something which has walking or swimming or some kind of tripping the light fantastic activity built in; think too about self catering so that at least you are in charge; or if breakfast has to be part of the deal, decide beforehand to give the fry ups a miss, and go for the fruit and more healthy options. Choose your favourite time of the day to have your most rewarding meal, and do *not* pick in between. If you must have ice creams, (Italy etc!) make it a *part of* the meal, or ensure you have enough activity to burn it off. Or stave off the best goodies till late, really late, in the holiday: "I've started so I'll continue", is frighteningly pervasive so the longer you leave it, the better. Conversely, if you are having a "go for gold" gastronomic holiday, do everything possible to "pay it forward" and shift a few pounds before going, and put a time line between coming back and going back to serious moderation. Many a stone is gathered from the holiday mode extending way past the return date. Draw a line in that sand!!

320

Mitigating circumstances...

There will always be... mitigating circumstances. You need to ask yourself whether there is a way out, whether you are excuse making, and how often the one off is – just that. Do you let yourself become embroiled in situations not of your own making, or is your life simply very eventful? Would you say you feel more or less in charge of your life, for the most part, or do you often feel more like a victim, acting somehow more at the behest of another than anything that truly represents your own nature? A look at the "big picture" and re-visiting what it is you actually want will again provide clarity for better decision making. If you feel your life, and hence your eating and your weight, is forever running round in circles, it may be useful to decipher how much of it is plain habit, how much is inevitable, and how much is perhaps pandering to the needs of others which may or may not be surplus to requirement. Emotional exhaustion can make coming off that hamster wheel almost impossible at times, but de-cluttering even tiny corners of your life, as discussed in Do, Delegate or Dump, can create a more than the sum of the parts freeing effect on your time, your energy, and hence your eating behaviours. Additionally, although I will not go into this here, a look at the social interactions between the psychological roles of victim, rescuer and persecutor in Stephen Karpman's Drama Triangle[58] might give you "food for thought"!

This is not about being genuinely vulnerable, genuinely supportive, or about anger which occasionally has a place and serves a purpose. It is rather when patterns of behaviour which typify one of these roles has a pay off which for our interests here, are playing havoc with your eating behaviours. The aim is to get wise to where we have become stuck in that triangle and to "step out".

Prolonged mitigating circumstances...

Should your "mitigating circumstances" be as prolonged as they are inevitable however, (this may include caring for an ill or elderly person) and should you have almost lost the plot with your eating habits, I cannot

---

[58] www.karpmandramatriangle.com

recommend enough that you get extra support whether by virtue of joining a group once a week, or if it's too difficult to get out, then by phone or Skype[59].

Psychologically, a change of perspective will probably be invaluable, and whilst I have largely left food itself out of the equation because it is so typically focussed upon to the exclusion of all else, the *kind* of food you eat really *can* help minimise cravings and help get you off the cake and carb trail before things go more seriously down, or uphill. It is not the rarest occurrence for the carer's health to deteriorate at some point, so caring for yourself to be well enough to continue optimal caring for the significant other, should hopefully be justification enough.

Keeping the Saboteur at bay!

More often than not, we are our own worst enemies! We sabotage ourselves at times with such sophistication, that as with the monkey who ate my breakfast, it can be as fascinating as it is infuriating or frustrating. *Be* fascinated however! When we are curious about ourselves, as opposed to condemning, it is our way to finding a way through and a better way of being, physically or otherwise.

Hopefully a lot of this book will have alerted you to the many sundry opportunities for your own sabotage, but for the moment, I want to flag up the kind of person who, consciously or unconsciously, sabotages you over and again:

Described in Karpman's "Triangle" as the Persecutor, a good example might be someone who knows full well you need to take care with your eating habits, yet always has temptation on offer. Refusal of whatever they have made "specially" may be met with a negative reaction, so you "rescue" them by complying. Being firm, not engaging with further discussion once you have reminded them of your intention, and not being swayed off your decision in response to their negative emotion will be the only way you will hold your ground. This does not mean you do not choose to indulge a person's need to have you eat the special whatever it is

---

[59] www.dietdetective.co.uk

they have made once in a while. It's becoming more aware when it is a repeated pattern which is in fact at your expense and offers you nothing except appeasing the other. While we are on the subject, you might also take note when reducing or normalising your eating whether the "persecutor" just happens to be you! Eating vicariously through the enjoyment of others is perfectly understandable and a common enough reaction but can be challenging for other overeaters trying to keep a balance! Just a thought!

Nearest and dearest and when not to say "no"!

It can be very disheartening for someone close to you to witness not only the ongoing saga of your struggle with food, and often as not to receive a lion's share of the blame, but to frequently be the one with whom you "go back to your diet". Assuming your partner, or whoever, really does have your best interests at heart, put your appreciation into action by factoring them in once a week, or once a month, in the eating stakes. If you have a reward day for yourself, make them *part of* it, better still, commit it to the Rolling Event Calendar so they *really feel* counted in! And if they *have* become a general scratch board for all ills, a receptacle for your sense of failure, let them know you realise this, and balance it a little at least by voicing your gratitude.

Knowing when to say "yes" to loved ones can make it far easier to say "no" the rest of the time, and make them far more supportive of your overall weight management.

Start with small steps and not with your head in the lion's mouth!

The ROLLING EVENT CALENDAR

All year long hundreds of occasions revolve around food or involve some kind of eating and drinking, directly or indirectly. While say the eight week period from early November to early January might be exceptional in the number of off the cuff or out of routine invitations, it is an excellent challenge in terms of testing out our ability to stay on track: it's also a great template for the rest of the year: Christmas for example, is only one day couched between a couple of Bank holidays including New Year, yet our indulging will often go from the first office social and roll on for the next thirty days! Throw in winter birthdays and whatever else and you can see what starts to happen. Your calendar will enhance your ability to *Pay it Forward* or *Return to Base* with increasingly nifty footwork on the days in between. Doing this enables you with minimal adjustment to maintain the safe weight of *Position One* (see Best Weight Safety Net and Window for Movement) and involves the kind of eating plan that is restrictive enough both in content and in calories to do its job, but tasty enough and filling enough to be tempting so you don't keep putting it off. We'll have a few examples in the chapter on food wisdom.

In contrast, events such as Ramadan have no days off in between a fairly extended period, and while abstinence from food and drink between sunrise and sunset might seem to work in favour of weight maintenance, it doesn't necessarily work out that way: there's invariably a lot of late night eating by way of making up and simply because one is over hungry by the day's end. Not going for gold, as I love to put it, on a nightly basis, as well as ensuring you have this in your year's Rolling Calendar, may incline you, more than at any other time in consideration of a whole month, to *pay it forward*, and to give your paying forward a definite date. Wrap it in a time frame!

* * *

Your 'Rolling Event Calendar' will always begin from today and extend for at least eight weeks ahead, on a rolling basis. This length of time is near enough to have relevance and not get ignored, and far enough ahead to still make plans.

The idea is that it will easily engage your attention so that at a glance, from day to day, you can see what is happening, and how your choices are leaving you with room to move, or not…

To this effect it needs to be simple, and it needs to be fun or at least hold your interest!! It particularly needs to be "in your face", so that you see it often, and so the contents, which you will add to most days, will always be somewhere in the periphery of your vision. Ideally it will then engage not just your conscious attention, but operate on a more subliminal, unconscious level as well.

Fill in all the social, work, and family events which are at all likely to involve food. Have a think and mark down on the calendar whether each of these are Easy, Not so Easy, or Challenging, and this might be with regard to logistics, i.e. where something is, or how long you've been up all day and how many or who will be there, or it might be an emotional issue, or because you will be tired after a long day or week. Note down in each square what the main challenge is. If particularly challenging, you might want to grade it 0 to 10.

Do take on board that "challenging" can just as equally include the mundane, or a lethal combination of everyday factors: for example, NOT succumbing to those biscuits left forever on view in the open plan office or place of work, whenever you have a dip in your energy levels or find yourself momentarily idle… added to not having had the sleep you need, or (ladies) time of the month etc, can be just as difficult as something more emotionally complex. Remember again your high risk combinations.

You might also colour code it accordingly: anything which will tell you with minimal effort how your next few weeks look. Yellow might be easier days, orange might be more challenging, and red or dark brown might bode disaster, but you get the idea.

Not only can you then see at a glance what you are up against, you will also notice whether you start to have far too many "challenging" events stacking up together. Often what doesn't seem difficult on days 1 and 2 starts to become an issue by day 4, if too many temptations or situations stack up together. It's the old, obvious, domino effect chestnut, except that obvious is never obvious enough. And if you think you know it well enough not to have to write things down, then ask yourself how come your eating behaviour shows otherwise... The idea is that if you keep falling down the same hole, over and over, this is a brilliant Up the Awareness, All Systems Alert activity which will require very little effort once you've set it up, and moreover help you clock those lethal combos or risk factors which bundle up together and trip us up, (see Putting it All Together and Identifying High Risk Combinations).

What also works well is to fill in retrospectively whether the level of ease or challenge was in fact as you suspected, or counter to this. If things don't pan out as you thought, it's information you need to remember, and this includes what went better than you could have hoped as well as the opposite. Have some gold stars ready to stick on if you successfully negotiate a difficult situation. A bit of self satisfaction goes a long way. That *is* the spoonful of sugar!

When you consider whether you are going to eat or overeat, think about whether it will be socially and emotionally valuable. Do you really want to renege on your goal for something which was really just an afterthought... Why put in calories which mean absolutely nothing, when they could be better enjoyed later on. It's like the choice between an enjoyable spend, or frittering money on rubbish and losing coins through a hole in your pocket wherever you go. If too, you become increasingly aware that you can't seem to stop eating or drinking, whether emotionally or just plain old habit, note that on your board as well. If you find you have quite an addiction going, sorting out what makes it worse is vitally important. This is yet another way of logging information so it's up there, in front of you. It's really no different to doing your accounts once a year. Even when you know perfectly well where the money's gone, the accumulated evidence can still be a shock!

FRAMING THE PROCESS and PRE-EMPTING DAYS *AWAY*...

Finally, to help "frame" the whole process and especially if you are going away, for work or for holiday, ask yourself:

What weight will be *fantastic* by the time I come back?
What weight will be *acceptable* to me by then?
What weight will be wholly *UNacceptable* to me?

This can be used equally for putting a "frame" around national or religious holidays: don't turn a day, or a few days, into a full blown eating season! Put it in a time frame.

Put something in place which will make drawing a line from holiday mode to "back in the zone", an easier process. Put it in the diary or on your calendar.

BE SPECIFIC!
Equally underpinning that:

What do I WANT...? What am I WILLING to DO...? What am ABLE to DO....?

Remember it is about *your* choice, setting *your* intention, and then keeping your eye on the prize!!

If this works well for you, you might consider doing a two month "roll" throughout the year. Doing this has two benefits: it really makes it much easier to keep an eye on what is going on, and doing it means you are serious!!

Have a look at the example calendar below, and then fill in your own.

Planning ahead is pivotal to successful weight management!

Rolling Event Calendar

Monday	Tuesday	Wednesday	Thursday	Friday	Saturday	Sunday
EASY! Day off work!	Dad's Birthday. Cake??	Work conference Sam rise - Paddington 6.45am	Work conference. long day plus travel back via main line station! CHALLENGING		Fitting for Lucy's wedding dress. Lunch with her friends...	Day off!
Auditing / Ofsted	Auditing / Ofsted	Auditing / Ofsted	work assessment results	In laws arriving for weekend. NEED to PLAN otherwise overtired. Could be challenging—		
DREADING	CHALLENGING	CHALLENGING	CHALLENGING	Hairdressers. Drinks with Jane and Lucy	Leave Sam!! Stanstead 7am. 5 hr flight CHALLENGING	
Reapplying for same positions at work - v anxious...		Prepare for holiday. Pack children's bags...Try NOT to keep picking!	Car service and MOT	TESTING		
Hotel Manager's Cocktail Welcoming party-		Sailing - lots of activity, but... a lot of eating / drinking temptation...				
Return home. 2 days off. Take-away tonight, then...	Moderating begins today! Lucy's wedding 2 weeks away. Great incentive...					

Etc etc...

COLOUR CODE: Easy / no problem – to slightly challenging – very challenging – high risk etc.

INCLUDE: Social / work / family events / domestic / emotional / physical / hormonal etc

INCLUDE: Plans to resolve, or planned ways around potentially difficult situations and times.

INCLUDE: Activities of all kinds – it quickly becomes obvious if you have too few!

INCLUDE: National as well as personal holidays. (You don't have to be celebrating a national or religious occasion to be tempted by adverts or extra food on offer....)

INCLUDE: *Anything* which potentially brings food or drink into the equation.

FACTOR IN / PAYING IT FORWARD: Whether a day, a week, or a longer period of time.

FACTOR IN: *Days off, or reward days* with partner, family etc, as and when appropriate.

					Monday
					Tuesday
					Wednesday
					Thursday
					Friday
					Saturday
					Sunday

REVIEWING the SITUATION: MOTIVATION LITMUS TEST

On the basis that motivation needs reviewing from time to time, this exercise is to help clarify some of the areas that could need your attention. When answering, think in terms of what you need right *now*, to get where you want to go!

You may want to spend more time on some of these than others. Before you finish, read through what you've written or reality check your assumptions. If you were listening to someone else telling you, would you be convinced? That's the litmus test for the litmus test!

What are you WILLING to do?
What are you ABLE to do?
What do you WANT to do?
What's your GOAL?
What's your MOTIVATION?
What might SABOTAGE you?

and

What are your HIGH RISK AREAS? These two may not necessarily overlap, but then again they might... Just think back over this last few weeks, what, (or who!) most threw you off course or prevented you getting back on?

What's your main, main reason for OVERCONSUMING? and I do not mean "oh it just tastes so good" or.. "pure habit". We're talking serious gremlins here...

and speaking of habit...

WHERE and WHEN?   have you been most likely to
fall by the wayside. The time
and the place. Habit thrives
on routine.

and conversely…

What kind of SITUATION?   most unsettles you and has led
in the past to eating more
than you need. To put it
delicately..!!

Note the use of past tense… to affirm a new start…
Yes…some of these questions are almost the same… just testing… but by
now hopefully you will be very clear about a lot of the answers!

WORKING THE SYSTEM...

"Paying it forward" in the way I've been talking about has been with regard to balancing your entire year. Stacking the odds in your favour so that more intense food moderation, when it needs to happen, is in harmony with other factors and keeps you ahead of the game.

Paying it forward at regular short term intervals works similarly. It may sound like yoyo dieting but the approach as well as the mindset is different.

We already know our propensity to reach for the reward of the here and now instead of waiting it out, is what makes dieting and long term weight holding so hit and miss: managing the minefield of social and emotional eating is about getting wise to the sheer abundance of triggers - tracing what lies beneath emotional overeating, and factoring in and working around those that stem from lifestyle. Somehow though, designed as we are for times of hardship to snatch what's available *now,* the old "instant versus delayed gratification" never quite goes away.

What other back up plan might we have then, to hold us to our resolve?

The answer is to factor that tendency *into* the equation.

Trying to be abstemious when you over use food in any way goes entirely against the grain so it's often a painful process. Interestingly though, there is seemingly far more difficulty **holding** to our hard won weight than actually getting there.

This works on the basis that we can just about manage to abstain completely from offending edibles, but find it far far harder to moderate once they're back on the allowance sheet! Proof of that pudding is the top favourite lie, "I'll only have one".

At the heart of much eating excess then is the silent beat of *either / or.*

The All or None reaction typifies the yoyo dieter so naturally, that surely implementing a mini version of this skill set into our efforts would make huge common sense! It's the psychological equivalent of vaccination where you use the hair of the dog, as it were, to immunise. Part of the poison *is* the protection, but you have to get the balance right!

333

So how might this be achieved?

I work with this in a couple of ways depending on whether you are wanting to lose weight, or hold your weight.

Current use of this premise is the 5:2 intermittent fasting plan (aka the Fast Diet[60]), or Alternate Day dieting[61]. Although both are used for weight *loss* I have found an adapted version of the 5:2 to work equally well for weight maintenance.

My only concern would be anyone whose overeating habits have too *much* of a hold, may find that on a weekly basis they are likely to keep deferring, so it never actually happens, or happens too rarely to be considered a valid weight watching plan. "I'll do it tomorrow / give this week a miss" catapulting you back into the same old trap where worse, you end up over indulging on the basis of the eternally imminent diet which is always about to begin.

For any kind of intermittent but regulated eating pattern to work, you have to know you can pull back the ropes, enough of the time. Again it is setting a routine, or a boundary in place, which becomes easier, with *habit.*

But the boundaries do *have* to work, *enough of the time.*

Other than this, it's a regime that only asks you to restrict the calorie intake two days a week and to quote Mimi Spencer, author of The Fast Diet - it's easy to comply and recalibrates the diet - so the odds are stacked in your favour.

Alternate day dieting, on the other hand, is a more extreme mini version of the All or None, stretched out over 48 hours. The reward is forever within reach, and not only does this offer sufficiently frequent respite but it imprints a delayed gratification habit in the process.

Whichever works best for you will depend as much on your efficiency in planning ahead as your ability to pull back the ropes.

Most people I have worked with prefer the 5:2 option, but as an inveterate overeater with issues round portion control, I find a gentler,

---

[60] The 5-2 Diet: Michael Moseley & Mimi Spencer / thefastdiet.co.uk
[61] The Alternate Day Diet: James B Johnson MD & Donald R Laub Sr MD.

middle of the road format for weight loss or weight holding is 4-2-1. Here's how it works:

Four days a week are the moderately lean days. No alcohol, processed carbohydrates or sugars, but you can still eat well. It's protein high, with an abundance of non starchy vegetables. Fruit if any tends to be berries... Come the 2 day part, in my case the weekend, by which time you've lost a couple of pounds with relative ease, the instructions are as follows: *Enjoy!!* Again speaking for myself here, by the day 1 bit, usually a Monday, I feel like I never want to eat as much again, so it works in my favour. This delusion lasts all of about twelve hours but sufficient time to use it to advantage and seriously cut back. That is the one *very* low calorie day, or protein and non root veg, and enough water to keep well hydrated.

This can be modified for weight *loss,* inasmuch that the "Enjoy" part of the equation would need to be curbed, whilst still allowing for larger portions and a "bit of a fix". I'll come to that though in the next chapter, on working the system with food.

The beauty of 5:2 and 4-2-1 for weight holding or weight loss is that they are not only workable, but *sustainable.* There is enough change so that you know you can hold to it most of the time. Alternating days if you prefer that option, has the reward forever within grasp, whilst 4-2-1 sandwiches the All bit between some of the None, and just enough of the "moderate" to hang in there while you perfect the practice!

It also incorporates the "nifty footwork" I mentioned earlier: the more skilled you get at hoppity skipping from one stage to another, the more you attain mastery over your eating.

Better still, when you do have times of excess, 5:2 or 4-2-1 are less likely to be eternally deferred, (with the weight gain that invariably takes place during a delayed deferment...) because they are *not* so radical. So whether the overloading has been pleasure driven or stress driven, once you have a period of calm, you can almost tip toe your way back in.

I am not suggesting for a minute that you do this if you are a naturally moderate eater. What would be the point? But for anyone whose need for a blow out has lasted a life time, this has within it a lot of what you need, with a little of what you want.

You *cannot* however, afford to delude yourself. As you practise the art of weight maintenance, and trust me, it is an art, you will find what works for you, or what works better, and what rarely works at all. But if you attempt the above and keep finding yourself stuck in the "All" bit, *Exit with Speed* and as soon as you are sufficiently settled, *Return to Base* and *Position One* and find something more workable for *you.* This is even more emphatically the case if you are in any kind of emotional maelstrom in which case ride out the storm till you can get your eating behaviours back into a relative state of normalcy.

BUDGET AND BANQUET!!

Budget and banquet works along the same lines, but as you might guess, this is not about losing weight, but maintaining what you have achieved.

There is little more wearying than towing the eating behaviour line for so long that a blow out *is* the only means to let up on the pressure. The problem with this, is that it's reactive rather than controlled. It features as frequently with people who are trying to lose just a few pounds as those who intend to lose far more, and the effect is often counterproductive. Many an escalation up the scales is borne of trying too hard to go down.

Because of this, Budget and Banquet works best on the premise that you already *have* a safety net, some window for movement in place, and that you are *able* to return to the budgeting. That safety net is not just about the physical weight, it's about your mindset, and once again, having *boundaries*. I use the word "budget" because it is no different to how we use money: the idea of a budget is not that you go wild and do irrevocable damage in the middle. If you are still out of control then your work may be about sorting something smaller, more immediately achievable than an eating regime which is still off your radar. Remember though, this is *not* about good or bad, or right or wrong: it's being realistic about how you *are.* However you feel, and whatever you may fear others are thinking, you are doing the best you can at any given time. That's *all* that matters.

I mention this now not to throw you off track, but because for so many, the "reward" of weight loss once it becomes the norm, is overshadowed by the prospect of lifelong restriction. Not surprisingly, there's trouble at mill soon enough and rebelling despite your best intent. Who wouldn't be with that kind of a mindset hovering in the back of your brain!

Rewarding yourself, appropriately, keeps you from chomping at the bit, feeling deprived and the inevitable outcome.

Wrapped in a time frame...

So budget and banquet is what it says but comes wrapped in a time frame, and ideally – it's planned. The 4-2-1 "formula", by way of example, comes with its own pressure release valve, i.e. the two days in the middle where you can go for gold, which means your need for let up is both given its due *and* contained.

Once again though, you need to have become deeply familiar with how you tend to operate and not play with fire. You may for example, want to *omit* foods that are serious triggers because that becomes less of a banquet and more of a **Red Alert Risk..!**

Banqueting is what you allow yourself when you know you can stop, and can "budget" with the more moderate eating on either side.

Because of this, it is useful to take care where and when you indulge. Do not choose times, or places, or companions which historically throw you back into old eating habits, where there would be an increased risk of not stopping.

Which means that the setting of boundaries, both in terms of a safety net weight window and a time frame, along with being realistic about foods that are red alert triggers, is what enables the reward in the middle.

a safety net weight window

Boundaries   =   *a time frame*

avoidance of red alert trigger foods or drink

Be mindful too, of **emotional boundaries** – which assumes an alertness to people and situations which have a trigger effect on your eating behaviour.

Taking on board – *please* – that none of the above is about bingeing or purging... there is often a fine line between addictive eating behaviours and simply having a terrific time, but you will get to know the difference. It will *feel* different, intuitively as well as physically. As you become adept at weight management, and by implication your eating behaviour management, you will become so attuned to your energy and how you are in relation to food, (though the ripple effect is far reaching into every area of your life...) that you will instinctively sense the difference between what is safe for you and what is a risk too far! Wisdom of course, is your ability to act on that insight and make choices that serve you well. The choice, is always yours.

Hopefully, knowing you will still be able to go gastronomically wild at times will brighten the horizon of your weight holding future!

TRICKS OF THE TRADE: FOOD WISDOM AND CURBING THE URGE...

I am not a nutritionist. I do however "walk my talk" so that as a woman of more than a certain age, I take care of my weight and wellbeing, and as a professional working with eating behaviours, I am authentic. This means that like a million other people out there, I know a lot about a whole variety of diets, but I also know what keeps me healthy and just how much I can play around with trigger foods and situations before things start to slip. Neither do I have a moral issue about weight or addiction: all I care about is that loss of control can take us to a terrible place mentally and physically, and that if we can hold a balanced relationship with food, we can find a way to enjoy ourselves without eating as a reaction to all and sundry.

My intention here is merely to provide a pointer in tapping your own existing wealth of knowledge, your common sense and your creativity with regard to discovering what works for you.

Throughout the book we have explored how eating behaviours are driven by emotions, by lifestyle and its many situations, and by variations in our physical wellbeing. The purpose, as I stated at the outset, has been to look at what despite so much effort to the contrary, keeps our faulty eating habits securely in place, other than the food itself which is the normal focus. Drs. Richard and Rachael Heller, founders of Carbohydrate Addict's Diet programmes describe the **triad of addiction** as comprising Behaviour, Environment and Biology, saying that in order to successfully correct an addiction all three factors in the triad must be corrected.

There is no doubt of the effect of stress, lifestyle, emotions and physical depletion on our eating behaviour and that many of those behaviours become habits. The effect of certain foods though in contributing to the vicious cycle of addiction, is equally without doubt.

My final port of call then before closing has to be a heads up with regard to very basic food wisdom: however much we address emotional or lifestyle issues underlying our overeating, we rarely find ourselves gaining weight with a profusion of apples or celery sticks. So what is it with the comfort foods and the starch and the sugar...?

Catch 22... not all in the head...

... carbohydrate *is* necessary for effective fat burning and to give us energy, but an *excess* can also be stored as fat in the fat cells. Additionally, too much *rich* carbohydrate causes your blood sugar to spike, which in turn causes your body to release too much insulin. This then causes your blood sugar to plummet, which sets off yet *more* intense cravings for *more* starch and sugar, because now the body wants to bring its blood sugar level back to normal, and those foods are the fastest way forward. What we get though is a vicious cycle impacting weight and health making us increasingly insulin resistant. As this gets worse, the recurring need for starch and sweets simply escalates. In other words there is a physiological susceptibility before you even start, so take a heightened insulin sensitivity, add emotional factors and too much or too little time on your hands, stir in habit over time, and you can see how we can really pick up that ball and run.

Eating excess (processed) carbohydrates ... leads to ...
increased blood sugar ... leads to ...
heightened insulin secretion ... leads to ...
more fat stored in your body cells ... leads to ...
low blood sugar, low energy, mood swing... leads to ...
more carbohydrate cravings ... leads to ...
eating excess carbohydrates ...

Over time, the combination of insulin increasing foods and emotionally or stress driven eating can create an imbalance of hormones that traps you into a catch 22 situation: the emotional eating starts to kick into gear even when the initial trigger is no longer there. The food itself creates more of the same and so it goes on.

340

In "The X Factor"[62], Lesley Kenton describes how ketogenics and insulin balance are key factors in weight loss, and keeping the weight stable. It's as good a guide as you can get. So where do we find the right foods?

How to break the cycle – the "miracle" crave busters!
Discovering which foods curb the cravings, together with practical tips for managing amidst the chaos go a long way toward healthy weight management! We *have* to keep our insulin levels in balance. Sugars, arguably *some* flavour enhancers, and complex carbohydrates like starch can all throw our insulin levels out of balance. Ultimately we need to find a way to work the system so we can eat well without overdoing it.

The low down is that whereas starch, sugar and foods rich in carbohydrates trigger an escalating insulin response and increasingly severe cravings, other foods have the opposite effect and genuinely curb the appetite.

For many, a sweet tooth is the downfall, whilst for others, dropping the wheat alone often has a transformative effect in reducing cravings, and dropping surplus weight, almost without effort[63] [64]. Such is the effect that many people, (I for one) will no longer have it as part of their staple food intake. The effort is more in letting *go* of anything wheat based over the first couple of days:

So the main questions will always be:

What kind of foods minimize the cravings?
What kind of food helps us to feel physically full?
What provides a substitute fix to feel emotionally and psychologically full, more of the time than not?

The above are not necessarily one and the same but on the basis of the obvious, that *feeling full is really helpful*, an exploration into the crave

---

[62] The X-Factor Diet by Lesley Kenton.
[63] Wheat Belly by William Davis.
[64] Wheat Belly Cookbook by William Davis.

curbing range of foods can be a revelation! Many of these come under the category of ketogenic foods. Briefly....

The Ketogenic range:
The type of foods which more easily *curb appetite* are high in protein and non starchy, non root vegetables, inducing the body to burn fats instead of carbohydrates. This does not mean an absence of carbs, which are needed to fuel the brain to function properly and provide energy to the body... but less of the over rich or processed variety which *over stimulate* the appetite.

Crave curbing protein:
Although not unique in burning body fat, the advantage of the ketogenic range of food, with protein such as meat, poultry, eggs, fish and shellfish, is that they help feel full more easily and help curb the cravings associated with consumption of *processed* carbohydrates, (aka comfort foods), more efficiently than anything else. Additionally some of that range including salmon, trout, mackerel, herring, tuna and sardines are rich rich rich in unsaturated, omega 3 fatty acids and are excellent for cardiovascular health and preventing heart disease.

Foods that are non starch or sugar, but fill:
Vegetables are an extremely important part of a healthy diet but the best for ketogenic purposes are dark and leafy, and anything that resembles spinach or kale will fall into this category. Similarly berries, kiwis and watermelon are better than more heavily fructose fruit such as apples and oranges.

This said, do your research online and take note of what works or doesn't work for *you!* Keep tabs on yourself as well with your "policeperson's note book" so you really do remember what you did before. An emotional "fix" which contains your eating can be just as effective, providing it does just that. When the body goes into what is known as ketosis however, it is possibly one of the best aids to weight management and gives willpower a massive helping hand. What I have found is that either keeping to a more ketogenic regime a few days of the week, or conversely , only having processed carbohydrates (i.e. bread etc) at *one* meal, really keeps the cravings to a minimum.

You do though need to take care should you be highly active, (I'm talking sporty active), that you are having *enough* protein, enough fluid and of course a balanced diet.

Foods that are ketogenic and... ready:
The *advantage* of supermarkets and the ready availables... is that we have everything we need in the appetite curbing range as well: at my busiest, some years back, I barely had time to think let alone eat properly, but I already knew that if I became over hungry it was a recipe for overeating disaster. At the ready in my kitchen pantry might be tins of sardines or mackerel, ham, chicken drum sticks, chicken slices, prawns, crab and other shellfish, baby corn, tofu etc. Eggs are in there as well, as is cheese in very small portions, as given more I eat the whole lot. If you can't be trusted, trust that you can't be trusted and shop accordingly.

Quality *and* quantity!
The great thing with ketogenic foods is that if you need to shift sharpish into weight loss, (either because of a sudden imminent event or because you've gone past a certain weight and more socially dodgy eating events are looming...etc...) there's nothing like a keto banquet on that first day to help still the appetite, stop the picking, and prevent going on the prowl for more food. Roast chicken does this a treat: it's a hit the spot item which fills the need for a fix gap. Ditto incidentally with cheese, which again may not be a good idea on a daily basis, but getting you past lift off can again hit the spot but curb further cravings. However if it's one of your *Red Alerts,* only buy a small packet or better still, don't go there.

And back to the conventional...

Uneconomical short term, worth the cost long term:
Give the buy one get one free items, or anything larger than required, as wide a berth as you can. Do not buy tubs of ice cream or whatever if either living alone, or with someone who is able to defer the temptation. As above, know when you can't be trusted and if you must have a high sugar or starch item, purchase the mini version, or two of the mini version.

FLUIDS! A *lot* of overeating is done when in fact we need fluid and have mistaken thirst for hunger: get used to carrying a small bottle of *water* wherever you go. If it won't "fit in the handbag" - unless you're out for the evening and in your gladrags – change the handbag! At the workplace make sure there is always enough available water for you to at least sip regularly. Many people say they forget – so set up reminders for you *not* to forget and create a new habit. It goes back to the "Do I value it enough" litmus test that shows you are still motivated, and committed to your plan! If you forget that easily, are you that serious?

Make sure too that you constantly have a 1 to 2 litre bottle near your desk. Any less and it's a faff to look for more when you're busy – and make this a habit over time, for the longterm, not just for a "diet".

Drinking enough fluid may not make up for all the deeply ingrained eating habits, but it will ***make a difference!***

If you know you drink too little because you find it too plain, you could add flavouring or try coconut water, (unlike coconut milk, very light in calories). Of course you can add some of the slimline or zero fizzy drinks but at least intersperse it with some normal fluid!

Foods that are quick to make:
Hate cooking? Too little time? Over hungry? Add your favourite minute to make menus to a little menu book.

Ideally you will have had something before stepping through the front door after work to keep the wolf at bay and curb the urge *enough*. If you are getting over hungry and going for too long without anything, you will need to break the pattern with something small which you can rely on having with you if you are out, or at work. Other than this, if yours is the hate cooking too tired category, make sure you have at least 3 to 4 menus a week that you either have defrosting, or really will take no more than fifteen minutes to make. Some people find using the crock pot or slow cooker, so that the meal is ready on arrival, really puts paid to the pre dinner picking episodes.

Example: Omelettes; cold chicken salad; tuna and light lemon mayo salad; avocado and tuna; avocado and egg... (all on the ketogenic list).

Tip: Ready made plain omelette cut into pieces and left in the fridge are great to combine with a quick salad. Alternatively eat on their own and accompany with a semi-skimmed latte to fill. Wait (or do something which will distract you...) 15 minutes and feel full!

Tip: Time to fess up! Having worked for a major weight loss company for over a decade, I have not only experienced the fantastic benefits of many of the nutritionally complete bars and food packs as an aid to ketosis, but found them one of the easiest, most convenient ways to maintain weight. Even one a day, when lack of time or planning might have made something more tempting and over high in processed carbs an all too easy option, means you don't get over hungry and you don't get over tempted.

The beauty of some of the bars is that they can be had in one, or cut into pieces and wrapped in cellophane to make taking one or two, as need requires, more likely; that they provide the much needed emotional "full stop" at either the end of a meal, later in the evening, or in the dangerous mid afternoon energy dip... *and* that they are ketogenic and taste good enough, without setting off the "must have more" brain change! Well, most of the time!

Equally the soup or shake packs are a wonderful lunch or late evening "comfort", whilst full of good vitamins and minerals. I am not ever suggesting that these are better than a conventionally balanced food intake, but they have the advantage of something quick yet replete when we lack time or imagination, and they keep the cravings at bay.

There are many out there online such as Exante, Boosch and Atkins though my favourites for taste include **Cambridge Weight Plan**, **SlimTuition**, **Ideal Weight** and **LighterLife**. Frankly in this day and age of rushed schedules and for anyone with a propensity to overeating, these are lifesavers!

You must however always ensure you get sufficient fluid intake with these and check with your GP before even attempting their sole use as a very low calorie diet (VLCD). This said, companies providing support for behavioural change in your relationship with food have good guidelines, together with strict medical protocol regarding foodpack consumption.

For anyone averse to the non organic, a totally natural alternative to this – in terms of providing a more personalised service - might be found with the aptly named Natural Ketosis Company[65]. Combining the convenience of the ready provided but with conventional food and support for your weight loss or weight management process, their website is worth a look.

Foods to take with you so you don't get over hungry:
These do *not* want to be too delicious or you might end up eating them before you are hungry. **As above!**

Foods that are *substitute fixes* and hit the right spot:
Once in a while you'll break the rules. Probably not an if but a when. But keeping that 1% in mind, there's a whole array of recipes that may not be everything you want but are a lot of what you need. They may not satisfy 100% but they get 75% of the job done, and the remaining percentage is more than made up for by the fact there's less craving.

Example: I am a double cream freak. Imagine my delight when I discover Lecithin granules, which emulsify the bad fats in your system, create a cream like as well as slightly crunchy effect when added to zero fat crème fraiche. Throw in some blueberries, (and if you're feeling utterly decadent a few drops of jus de cassis for good measure...) and it seriously does the trick! No it *isn't* the real thing, but providing I can "banquet" once a week for weight maintaining, I can live with that.

Example: Avocado and baby corn salad. Add ham, bacon bits or the quorn vegetarian equivalent for extra "hit" and mix with virgin olive oil. Yes it is high in calories, but as with the dessert above, it's good, it's healthy, and because it hits the spot, I'm not overeating or picking later on. I'm done in one!!

Tip: Researching the vegetable / olive oil range and investing regularly in

---

[65] www.naturalketosis.co.uk

your favourite really brings life to the blandest of dishes. Additionally, herbs such as fresh ginger and grow in the pot coriander, parsley and basil give a hit that is emotionally filling as well as great for the system!

Example: Instead of a latte and especially when the weather is hotter, add something like one or two heaped teaspoons of organic cold milled flax seeds, to a glass of non soya Almond Alpro. A great source of fibre, protein and omega 3, it is lightly sweet so its effect as a cold drink is to fill, to hit the spot, *and* keep you regular – often a problem when dieting. Alternatively sprinkle a generous tablespoon of milled flax seeds and goji berries on yoghurt or oats.

Tip: Again depending on your aim – i.e. banquet day or weight loss /weight holding etc - a range of minute to make or already made sauces can transform an otherwise "sensible" meal into a hit the spot winner: on the moderating front – I have a stack of 0% fat fromage frais which I add to spices, steamed mushrooms, tomatoes, cucumber - which combined with fish or salad or poultry or bundle loads of steamed green veg are wonderfully palatable and work a treat on budget days. I round off with a "full stop" and rarely feel deprived. Providing you don't torture yourself with too many food ads and cooking shows!

Alert: Caution with the "lower fat" categories: they often have a heightened sugar content to make up the taste.

Foods that are *full stops:*
This may vary according to whether it's one of your banquet days, a budget day, and whether you are holding a weight you are happy with, or aiming to lose weight.

This is anything which irrespective of whether you are actually hungry or not, and let's face it at the end of a meal no one is genuinely *hungry,* provides a psychological *stop.*

It could be at the end of a meal, but it could also be a mid afternoon pick me up which does the job and is self containing. The operative word is *self containing!* Whether it's a fruit, a single coffee, a piece of cheese, a piece of chocolate or an Atkins / LighterLife / Cambridge type bar to finish off - it's small, and the idea is it rounds off the eating. If habitually it has the opposite effect, then it ain't a fix or a full stop. It's a red alert. Know the difference. Know what works.

Tip: Don't count the calories, as the calories these are saving are the ones you're not picking at later on. That's why they work.

Listen to your body.

Notice what fills you, and notice what satisfies you emotionally. Many overeaters can have a great meal, but if it doesn't hit the button, the mind is on the prowl.

Rule of thumb on budget or management days*:

- Cut *out* wheat, starch, gluten, sugar.
  Which means no processed carbs such as bread, cake and biscuits, no root vegetables such as potatoes and parsnips, and no sweets or sugar drenched drinks.
  (*The exception to this may be diets such as the Carbohydrate Addicts Diet[66].)

- Make your main meal of the day **at *least* 20 minutes long**. (That really isn't much but it allows for non social eating and when your day is one long rush.)

- Make sure it has something you can **crunch and munch** on.

- Make sure it has something which is a substitute *fix*. If you're an emotional eater or food is your reward – the monkey mind is likely to be on the prowl for extra goodies unless it's had that fix.

---

[66] The Carbohydrate Addict's Diet: The Lifelong Solution to Yo Yo Dieting by Dr Rachael F Fuller & Dr Richard F Fuller.

So that's a 20 minutes minimum, a crunch, a munch, and a hit the spot fix...!!

Food categories for *you* – i.e. allowable - to not worth the risk:
Food triggers… allowable to not riskable… i.e. in my case - bread. Alcohol for the alcoholic. Etc. Once in a while I have amazing bread when I am outside of the home. But I notice I am thinking about it for days after. Take note, use your common sense and give danger zones a wide berth:

Know your RED ALERTS list:
Bread and butter. Cheeses. Ben and Jerry's chunky monkey ice cream. Anything which feels like there's a chemical brain change going on..!! Don't go there! Don't pretend it's for someone else if the someone else always ends up being you. It might be endearing, but it isn't funny. Clear your kitchen where possible of anything which acts as a brain changing trigger and pretty well only gets eaten by you. If your partner would like the food "some of the time" and you have a serious weight issue, get him or her to keep it somewhere out of sight.

If the person is a child, check whether they really need it, or are you nurturing the same bad habits in your beloved offspring? If they get demanding, remember, it's *your* health, and you're in charge. It's not a democracy when you're paying the bills – *you're* the boss! By the way we're not talking unhealthy food restriction here and focus on dieting, so much as leaving out junk foods that generations before wouldn't have *been* in the house! You won't create an anorexic child by not buying surplus crisps and snacks and sugars. By contrast, if you're forever yo yo dieting, you really are bringing attention to food and weight issues. Teaching by example, that is by what you actually *do* rather than what you say, is a great incentive to following a healthy eating regime, and keeping your weight stable.

Hiding the Red Alerts!
Unless you live alone, and possibly even then, there is always likely to be something which falls into this category hanging dangerously around, waiting for temptation to ambush as resolve weakens. (Note I am giving

them a will of their own but that is how it can feel!) Find a place they are hidden from view or more difficult to reach. That's up high, on top of and at the back of the cupboard or frozen at the back of the freezer. Our brains respond to visual cues, so out of sight is good! It may not work all of the time but it will work some of the time and that is a place to start.

Not cooking the Red Alerts!

I haven't come across any experiments conducted in the above but my own sense is that steaming or baking is far less likely to titillate the taste buds than frying. Check out your own response (again, collect the evidence to negate selective memory!) but if you find this to be the case, steam, bake, grill, microwave... just leave out the fry up!

Creating your *own* menu book:

One of the delights of creating your own menu book and lists of recipes, is that over and above being able to recall at a glance what works for you over time, and in different situations... (tiredness and stress for example creating different needs), is that it doubles as a "filling the gap" project. It can be a distraction in itself.

Along with conventional recipes that you enjoy and work for you, it's useful to include your lists of:

"Hit the Spot" and **"Hit the Spot *Fast!*"** items.
"Substitute Fixes"
"Need for a Fix" gap fillers.
"There in a moment ready mades" and other quick to make recipes.

Equally, include your favourite "diets" that work for you. Depending on circumstances, timing, how you're feeling and what you're actually aiming for, you will find different approaches work at different times. Rule of thumb again however, is ***Don't mix the diets!!*** Unless you have become queen of diets and really know what you are doing, (which you might), mix and match is more likely to confuse, and is rather like mixing maps and wondering why you keep getting lost!

350

MENU PLANNING:

If you are remotely able, planning for the week *ahead* means that to a greater extent, as soon as you come back home, you can focus more easily on the job in hand and not find your mind on the prowl. It does rather assume you have enough in to cater for this, and that you have planned as equally for the shopping at an earlier point in the week. It might also be that in order to accommodate this even three days a week, before you fall off your perch with life and other issues, you may have to err on the side of simplicity, but this is a time when deliciously dull can work in your favour long term.

Eating Out! Create your best restaurant list:

It may not always be up to you, but if you are able to choose a restaurant you are at least better informed before the start:

By way of example – sometimes I will choose a French restaurant because I know the portions *are* smaller! Or I know if I go to Pizza Express there are several dishes which, providing I ask for the doughballs *not* to be brought, are tasty but ketogenic. So I can eat out, have tasty food *and* keep things contained! (But must keep my beady eyes off other people's dough balls....!)

For the long term, create a ***regime*** rather than a diet:

A regime as a way of *being* can embrace both moderation as well as a love of food.

Eating Behaviour Recognition:

Unsure as I am where this best fits since it is as much about mindset as food, I have opted for here on the basis of, hopefully, greater relevance...

Over the years I have noticed not only a propensity to mix and match diets which at times might be best left apart, but an equally strong inclination to boomerang from one state of reactive eating to another: possibly the hyperactive eating behaviour equivalent of the French general who famously mounted his horse, and rode off in four different directions at once, the outcome is often despondency, yo yo dieting and more mental torment. So. Below is the nearest I can describe in type, to a train track of eating pattern station stops.

Recognition: Getting to know the road and train track to success...

Overeating /
  Drinking...
    Normal Eating
      i.e. a Balanced intake
        Reduced Calorie / Lower or Low Calorie Diet (LCD)
        Your own version or
        WeightWatchers or
        Slimming World, whatever...
          Generous Ketogenic / Fast Fat Burning LCD
          Strict Ketogenic / Fast Fat Burning LCD
          Total / Very Low Calorie Diet (VLCD)
          Ketogenic / Fast Fat Burning...

Rather than having to boomerang from one extreme to the other, your train track enables going back or forward in easier stages. Where it comes into its own, is if you have slipped and can't quite get back on the straight and narrow, or if a change in schedule necessitates a small but more subtle shift in what you'd previously intended. It's another branch between the extremes of All or None to enable balanced thinking and better weight management.

Ultimately, the aim always is that instead of having to resort to others for advice about dieting, *you* will become your own best counsel. After all, no one else will have the necessary information on yourself to make the best decisions. The more you familiarise with your ***own eating behaviour blueprint***, the more you will be your ***own most trusted guide***.

Checking the food labels:

Part of *becoming* your own "most trusted guide" will not only include greater mindfulness with regard to your eating behaviours, and how they happen, but equally becoming more vigilant as to what is actually *in* the food that you choose to buy. Most canned, tinned or packet foods nowadays have pretty distinct labelling with regard to content, so you can no longer claim ignorance! Becoming informed enables far better decision making, and you might just decide that that 500 calorie pork pie filled to the brim with fats and all sorts, may not seem so attractive after all. Leastways not on a regular basis.

Tip: Take yer specs!

Useful too to get in the habit of taking your reading specs if required: some of the ingredient and nutrient listing is *awfully* small!

* * *

Assuming you have had ongoing issues with your weight, and depending on how heavily this is driven by any one of the issues we have looked at throughout the book, your driving question will again be:

Which bit of the combined matrix of lifestyle and circumstance, emotions, physical wellbeing and food itself will be the easiest bit to change first?

It can be a one off, tiny tiny change, appropriate to the day, the time, whatever you are doing and how you are feeling that particular week.

It can be a change that varies over time, according to what fits in and works best for you: whether it's a better night's sleep making you less susceptible to comfort snacks, better planning so you never shop when you're hungry, a shift in the food itself or if you're on top form, then all of the above!

Whatever you choose, my recommendation would be to look at the practical first. It is tangible and so will usually be the easiest to address and repair. Then you can tackle the emotional. But go with your instincts on this. If something doesn't work for you then you're the one in charge and you can change it. Nothing is set in stone except for your commitment to an easier, healthier way to eat well, stay healthy, and avoid foods which create too much craving.

Knowing that you can make any number of "first small steps" at any given point will lessen the pressure, the frustration, and the likelihood of yet more carb to quell the angst!

In order to make it easy however, you will need to implement some kind of routine so you don't have to keep thinking about it. The problem simply gets put to the side when it takes up too much head space in an already busy schedule or if we're feeling down or badly need a reward. This is where your increased awareness of how you operate, how and when your eating tends to get affected, enables far better choice making about what you are doing and the food you choose... and just in *case* you are thinking you are fine when on form, my question would always be – and how often is that?

My own experience is that while I work well enough most of the time, fact is my stress levels range from slight to considerable at any given time bar days off or on holiday - and the temptation to reward with just a little of something here and there all too easily adds up. So you make plans on how you are *as a rule*, not on some fairy tale version of how your imagined ideal would be. Great to aspire toward, but not to be relied upon for practical planning. What you rely on is the composite information derived from the information gathered thus far, be it with ongoing variations as and when necessary.

So for anyone who over enjoys their food, or who over compensates with food, **planning and preparation** is beyond pivotal to the plot. Somehow not managing this means you either still don't get the significance so you just don't prioritize it into your day, or you have difficulty schedule wise or emotionally accomplishing the task and one or both of those still needs re-examining. Again, it isn't about right or wrong or being good or bad, it's about **recognition and remembering** - which is where your **Rolling Event Calendar** comes so beautifully into its own.

Remember that **timing...** which we looked at already in Budget and Banquet – will help provide those new boundaries which in themselves become the kind of habits we *need* to have. As those habits settle in and override the older non helpful ones, that already will start to shift the momentum of healthy eating and hence healthy weight management in your favour. Installing a new, small habit in this respect even once a month is all it needs, and will work wonders.

Be active! Do research that at once strengthens your resolve *and* puts that Automatic Pilot working in the direction you need!

The more you increase your already existing wealth of dietary and food for health knowledge, the more you add to your expertise, and own best judgement - *and* the more it all filters through into that behind the scenes part of your brain, insuring the good habits take charge, instead of an automatic impulse that rarely works in your favour! (aka Automatic Pilot / bad habit / Wild Monkey at the wheel / not your rational self etc ....!!)

The books I have listed below however are some of my well used stand bys over time – the first three especially providing easy to read information about the biological mechanics of weight gain, but there is a fantastic list of blogs out there to add to your daily repertoire of life and health enhancing menus for the ever increasing weight watching millions! Or you might take time browsing through the shelves of your local health shop – discovering new foods that are at once a substitute fix *and* a health boost has to be a great way of *minding that gap!!*

The more you take care of the cravings, the more the calories take care of themselves!!

Further Reading

"The Carbohydrate Addict's Diet: The Lifelong Solution to Yo Yo Dieting" by Dr Rachael F Fuller & Dr Richard F Fuller

"The South Beach Diet Cook Book" by Dr Arthur Agatston

"Living Lighter Lite – Lighter Life: Life in Balance Recipe Book"

"Meals in Minutes – Cambridge Weight Plan"

PART 6: SUMMING UP

SUMMING UP

There have been three times in my life when my eating behaviours took a sharp shift in notably different directions: the first, a year or so into my flying career when fatigue plus ever available eating opportunity took its toll, saved only by vanity and the proximity of hotel pools and gyms. I know, lucky for some, but it took consistent effort to bring the two and a half stone back into line in order not to waddle uncomfortably at altitude. On the days I succumbed, badly, I am all too aware looking back, of the eternally present jet lag which exacerbated an already existing propensity to over enjoy food!

The second was a welcome if unexpected moderation, just days into my first visit to the Findhorn community in Scotland. Overjoyed as I was with the home grown food, the pantry shop that you could just sign your name and pay later, the presence of freshly made bread on offer late evening and the all inclusive three meals a day and some - I stuffed myself so shamefully that by day three, the final venture into some new tofu variation had such intestinal impact, I was sure my imminent demise would say, "died of greed." Predictably, shock would have incurred a day or two of necessary restraint, but to my surprise it continued then and on each return visit for many years. What I realised, when it finally dawned on me, was the intensity of happiness and emotional nourishment was far different from anything I had previously experienced. One might muse that in searching I had "found myself" but the point remains the same: something had settled and the eating had gone down a notch.

The final, more recent shift, was my third year visiting a friend in the French countryside. Concerned at the reappearance of old eating habits as increasingly long visits prolonged the inevitable holiday dining mode, I returned early summer to find the potager he'd begun in the spring was producing an abundance of vegetables. Domestic goddess, not, I have never in my life cooked beetroot and certainly not one the size of a football, but the result, along with a profusion of potatoes, parsley, tomatoes, broccoli and rhubarb... together with an uncommonly prolific amount of fruit from nearby trees giving us figs, cherries and walnuts, meant we dumped getting meat or fish for the duration and lived off the land. Knowing where the food came from was manna from heaven and felt, dare I use the word, sacred. Something in the order of things felt balanced, and exquisitely once again, moderation followed.

So Charlotte Hofton's statement that obesity is rarely about greed[67] has my wholehearted agreement. Already a proponent of the "body as messenger" school of thought, I see it merely as a warning light that something is out of harmony. Whether that lack of harmony or dis-ease is mundane or complex, whether it is from a single source or a combination of factors creating mayhem, you will always be your own best judge and only you can make the necessary choices. It may feel like deprivation but to paraphrase Julia Havey in her book The Vice Busting Diet[68], the only real deprivation is limitation on your lifestyle and sense of self. Obesity is not a lifestyle choice: it is more usually a prison sentence doing damage to your body and any sense of personal accountability.

Resonating my own sentiment, Hofton concludes her article suggesting that a doctor's first question should not be "How much do you weigh?" but "How unhappy, tired, wretched, impoverished, isolated or in pain are you?".

Hopefully, many of the questions in *this* book will spark, if not an epiphany of recognition, then enough lightbulb moments to waylay that untimely doctor's visit and help some of you take action *before* the fact. Freedom, as I said at the outset, is not merely permission to taste the forbidden, but the ability to say "no" when we choose. Without this we are simply slaves to our senses with the frightening consequences already in so much evidence.

On a lighter note, and to consolidate the recognition that Overeating Unplugged has as its aim, I will leave you with what I believe to be some of the finer points of weight management and a set of golden rules! More importantly however, since the greater quest is for you to become your own best detective, add your own whenever they come to mind.

---

[67] Charlotte Hofton: Isle of Wight County Press: 04/04/2014.
[68] Julia Griggs Havey: The Vice-Busting Diet.

Participate in establishing your own brilliant Eating Behaviour Blueprint and enjoy the journey!!

Finally, in a last attempt at minimizing the "it's not fair" pattern of thinking, remember that if your overeating has taken you too far up the scales, your new eating regime is less to do with dieting and more about bringing your eating back to *normal*. Just a detail, I know, but the word diet is so laden with connotations. Food for thought!!

Diets are temporary bridges from one place to another:
A regime is for life and a new way of being.

The Dynamic of Opposing Intentions.
Or the 1% seesaw principle and variations on a theme

1 You have to *want* what being slimmer will *give* you, 1% more than the *extra* food / drink (if you've achieved your goal weight and are maintaining) *enough* of the time.

I'm saying *enough* both because that really is all that is necessary *and* I'm not giving anyone a foothold into the must be perfect / all or none / obsessive pathway to "I've blown it".

2 "I've blown it"... and adaptations on this theme, (check out your favourites so you familiarize with what to look out for and eventually avoid..) is singularly *the* most fattening thought process there is. Ok, it possibly follows on from "I'll die if I don't have that doughnut" or "I'll be darned if I don't have that doughnut", but these are still aspects of Distorted Thinking.

3 There is a gap between Intention, i.e. what you decided you were going to do first thing in the morning, and Behaviour, which is what you actually end up doing, as a rule, by the end of the day. All overeating or drinking, (or smoking or anything in fact) has a function, and that is, in some way, to Fill a Gap. It might be filling the gap because you need bits of structure to separate out your time, like a pause, or a full stop here and there to give yourself a break or mark a moment, or it might be to provide stimulus, and entertain yourself in some way, to alleviate boredom, or to defer some task, some event. Or it might be a way of coping if emotions are uncomfortable and cause distress.

But if what you Mean to Do and what you End up Doing are forever at variance, and if that is now jeopardising health and peace of mind and taking up a lot of your time, you may as well start deciding how to Mind the Gap, instead of filling it.

Intention	*Filling the Gap*	*Behaviour*

← ————————————————————————————————— →

What I said I'd do	*Filling the Gap*	*What I actually did*

What you need is to start noticing all the things that contribute to the variance. Before you do anything, and assuming this is important enough to you, recognition is key to checking whether you really want this.

Minding the Gap

Recognition is the key	*Filling the Gap*	*Motivation is the fuel*

What usually goes wrong is that consciously or unconsciously, we have loads of other things that are fighting for the same level of prioritization.

It's like having two conflicting destinations. Say Hampshire and Scotland. Let's say getting slim is Scotland, (choose your own) and all the old routines and habits with everything that constitutes those routines and habits and takes you astray is Hampshire.

4 At every moment, you are either heading toward Scotland, or Hampshire.

This will be evident in your actions, but your thoughts come first, whether in awareness, or out of awareness. Scotland or Hampshire... Scotland or Hampshire.

5 Your job, initially, is simply to notice the thoughts that keep taking you back to Hampshire, or if things are especially dire, keep you from even leaving Hampshire. (Yes, I am serious.) Just notice, observe. Then start to jot them down. Make a record of them.

It's a bit like a magician pulling a scarf through a hole. If you can just grab hold of one end, you can pull it all the way through. But you need to decide you want it and keep focussing until you've pulled it all the way through.

6 The Dynamic of Opposing Intentions tends to produce confusion and doubt.

Your job is to check out what these could be, and start, if your motivation is genuine, to rearrange them in line with your most heartfelt aim.

Being unsure, or wanting things which cancel each other out or conflict in some way, produces conflict and usually sends you back the wrong way. Conflicting desires set up a struggle.

A *settled decision* will not only give you peace of mind, but take you to your goal.
Recognising the stuff that is in conflict, however minimal, is the *first step*.
Recognising that you have, or don't have the *motivation* saves time money and energy.

Motivation is the fuel   *Settled Decision*

——————————————————————————————➤

Recognition is the key   *Laser like focus*

As Pam Grout tells us in her wonderfully, out of the box book[69], "If your mind is engaged in an ongoing showdown between different, conflicting parts of yourself these splintered intentions set all sorts of dynamics into motion".

7 Keep your eye on the prize. Remember the difference between what you *actually* want, and the gratification of a whim. Think about things you have achieved, whether with innate ease, or in the face of a challenge: your thoughts and actions would have had sufficient momentum to pull you through, like the scarf, through that "hole" and up to fruition. Your focus would have been one pointed, laser like, in its aim. Lasers have wavelengths of only one size, which lends them pinpoint precision.

—————————————

[69] "E-Squared: Nine Do-It-Yourself Energy Experiments That Prove Your Thoughts Create Your Reality" by Pam Grout. Hay House Insights 28/01/2013

Intentions that are focused are integrated like a laser, with a single, clear beam.

8 The abiding question is always:

What do you Want?

What are you Willing to do?

What are you Able to do?

Hampshire or Scotland... your thoughts and actions will take you backwards, or forwards.

Realising what you've been up to all along, the choices you have been making in or out of awareness is *the* first step.

Rearranging those choices in a way that is in line with your ***Main Choice, IS your choice***. It is up to you.

9 Being Unconscious of the underlying dynamics and thoughts and actions, or for that matter, not attending to the obvious and not always so underlying is like leaving your house in charge of a bunch of children for a week and wondering why it is all such a mess and what could possibly have gone wrong. Getting to grips with the situation helps you decide what to do and to know whether it is possible. But awareness, becoming conscious, comes first. Realising what you're doing, and realising what you're thinking that's leading to the doing is totally pivotal to the plot.

So when and why you keep eating or drinking is as crucial as what you are eating.

10 Don't assume you'll remember.

Your final step in this section is to *not* assume you can remember this, or that it is obvious.

If it were that obvious, you'd be in charge of all your eating behaviours and not have a problem in the first place. Anything which provides insight is best recorded, written down someplace. Remembering the obvious is the domain of the rational mind. Most of this operates on a different level.

It's an automatic impulse, otherwise known as unconscious behaviour, which has a pull and a will of its own. It's the bit of you which, in awareness, abdicates on a whim and undermines all previous good intent. Out of awareness, well, you don't even know it's happening till after the fact.

What you're collecting is the evidence of any thoughts or actions that take you away from your goal.

11 PRIVATE INVESTIGATOR... In order to lose the weight and hold that weight at the right end of the scale, you will need to become your own best private detective and *notice* what you are up to at any given moment.

The case you are onto is your own. Think C.S.I. (Crime Scene Investigation unit).

The devil is in the detail. Each of you has your own Eating Behaviour blueprint.

Recognition of this has to come first. Think When, Where, Who, then Why and how come.

Why and how come include the feelings and thoughts that underlie the impulse, which combined with the rest, create varying degrees of that powerful impulse to lapse, or do what you did before!!

Be curious, rather than angry or disappointed or upset: being upset simply creates reactive behaviour more often than not (Rebellious Child...) and guess what we often do to comfort ourselves..! It rarely serves the purpose we want and takes us back to Hampshire!! Follow your trail of behaviour. Be delighted with each new insight, each lightbulb moment, and take small steps, day at a time.

12 CAMERA CREW "Big Brother 24/7" To put the proverbial dot on the "i", imagine a nationwide slimming version of "Big Brother". Everyone knows your aim is to change your eating and drinking behaviours and lose weight, but there is no sound, and we are not privy to your thoughts. All we can see is what you are actually doing at any moment in time. Ask yourself, would it *look* like you were trying to get slim? What would we actually see?

Alternatively if it were "Jo Frost Supernanny" watching on the webcam, what would she see, and what might she say? Remember she is never shaming, simply instructive.

Have fun!

Ps: I have nothing against Hampshire!! I simply chose two opposing ends of the country!

Golden Rules of Successful Weight Management
...and staying light!!

Taking pride of place:

- *If you do what you did before, you'll get what you had before.* Leaving out more often than not whatever took you up the scales, may feel like a diet, but it isn't. It's eating ***normally.***

- **The Energy Equation - Weight *Loss*:** the more out, than in, rule. If you're aiming to lose weight, there needs to be a deficit. You might eat less, eat differently, or move around more, but somehow or other there needs to be more calorific energy burnt off than taken in.

- **The Energy Equation - Weight *Maintenance*:** as above, except you're aiming for stability. There needs to be a balance, often enough, over time.

- **The Energy Equation - Your individual Energy Expenditure:** Check the calorific output for your weight, height and general activity level. This will go down as you lose weight, but provides your framework.

- ***Planning is pivotal:*** There's an old adage that says "if you fail to plan, you plan to fail". Grating, but usually true. Your best chance of overriding that automatic impulse and unconscious habit, is with military precision, and **planning**!! Should you forget, which is normal some of the time, "How come I *forgot* to plan" will give as much information as "how come I overate".

- ***Notice*** what you do. Be alert, observe. Befriend rather than berate and use lapses or cravings as ***information.*** Like the ***red light*** on your car dashboard they register imbalance, however slight. Notice when, what, who, why etc.

- ***Collect the Evidence*** and keep a record. It's your ***detective in action!!*** Know more and more what works for you.

- ***Red Alert - avoid shopping when tired, stressed or hungry!***

- *Boundaries - No picking between meals!* Apart from "retraining you", this gives the digestive processes a rest between meals, hence reducing over time the old "food calls".

- *Red Alert - "Uncountables" are unaccountable!!* Packets of nuts or raisins and suchlike are wonderful side bits to go with drinks or at any time of the day but it's all too easy to lose sight of how many you've had, or simply not want to stop. Plus they pack a calorific punch. Have only one small packet at a time to hand!

- *Timing - Do not eat large and late as a rule...* The debate always rages but common sense surely applies: there's little energy expenditure with eating a large or heavy meal shortly before you retire, hence, adding to weight issues: acid production can contribute to reflux while lying down, undigested food is left to ferment, and the body doesn't rest as fully. When possible, finish eating a good three or so hours before turning in, but if you have no choice or you need that "full stop", make sure it is light.

- *Timing Do NOT get over hungry!* Too long a stretch without food means you run the gauntlet between leaving work and getting home, or at any time when being too hungry and the need for a treat kicks in big time! The two of them in tandem are terrible. *Keep the wolf from the door* with a *planned* mid afternoon (*non* trigger) snack, or at least an hour or so before you leave work.

- *Timing Wait 20 minutes after eating!!* If you can factor this in or find anything to distract you elsewhere, the brain finally registers you are full and makes it less likely you'll keep returning for more!

- *Eat slowly, chewing the food well!* Apart from giving us longer to actually *feel full*, chewing more thoroughly creates a food / saliva mix which breaks it down more easily and enables a better release of nutrients.

- *Sitting down to eat* helps us make the most of our meal even if it's only 15 minutes! Getting in the habit of making our eating time emotionally valuable will highlight all the more when we're eating mindlessly. So by implication do **NOT** as a rule eat on the run / on the sly / in the car / standing up etc.

- **NO bogofs! (buy one get one free..) No "economy buying"** if it's a *false economy!* Buy one get one free works wonderfully if the number of freebies or extra portions matches your family number. If you're paying over time for one diet or another, that minute in the mouth / month on your hips will outweigh any savings and exact a far greater emotional cost. Do not even go there.

- **Read the food labelling!** - Get wise to calorific, nutrient and food content.

- **Leave trigger foods in the shop or out of sight** If you have a serious problem with a particular food, why go there? If it's "for the rest of your family", make sure it's the case! Trust when you can't be trusted!

- **Foods between the ALL or NONE** Have your list of **non trigger "fix it" foods** which enable Return to Base or Position One! Some people jump in, others need to tiptoe almost tricking themselves back into the zone. Again, whatever works for you.

- **Full Stops** Know what acts as a "full stop" on your eating. It's usually less to do with hunger and is more about a change in taste and emotionally "rounding off" your meal.

- **Weigh yourself at least once a week!**

- **Make Returning to Base a Habit!**

- **Maintain your Safety Net with window for movement!**

- **Factor in an annual MoT (Motivation over Time!)** It is normal for complacency to grow and motivation to slip. Factor it in by reviewing your eating patterns, activity levels, and lifestyle "choices", at least once a year, and ideally on a monthly basis. Time spent takes care of the pounds or the kilos. Count it in as you would any commitment you were serious about. Put it in your diary, your phone, your Rolling Event Calendar.

- *Maintain Movement - as in "anything up from zero" is better than none!* Find any way you can to keep active. It doesn't matter what! It burns calories, works the body and puts you in virtuous mindset!!

- *Devise tactics for portion control Buy less, make less!* If at first you don't succeed, squirt leftovers with washing up liquid and chuck them in the bin - fast!! If this appals you, all the better: your discomfort will make you think twice before the surplus buying or cooking.

- *Maintain your best practice when calm (enough)* It is normal for a lot of the old habits to return as a "job lot" when the going gets tough and you're on an emotional or situational rollercoaster. For this reason alone, do your utmost best when the waters are calm and whatever constitutes your general environment is less demanding.

- *Use your common sense and intuition* It tells you a lot! *Be honest with yourself. Taking responsibility* in this way is the primary route to genuine self care. Remember, you are your own *best expert!* If it works for you, it works for you. That's all that counts.

- *Listen to your body* As per above, it tells you a lot. If you have been overeating and hence overriding your body's signals for a long time you may never get hungry enough to notice. Once you revert to balanced eating the signs, which might include a sensitivity or intolerance to wheat, gluten, sugar etc, will be there. Notice too what energises as much as what depletes.

- *Know your psychological and emotional horizon* I.e. What's on the forecast? Again get to know your signs and get to act on them. If you find you tend to underestimate the effect of something on your eating, keep collecting the evidence till you can rely on your accuracy, enough of the time.

If you feel an "attack" coming on, learn to recognise whether it's a passing urge or a big time craving. Rollercoaster cravings and eating binges don't generally arrive unannounced, however much it might seem that way. They have usually taken anything from a few hours to several days to fully develop. Learn to recognise the signs with whatever conditions bring them on and prepare as best you can.

- *Always start with easy* - Small, totally achievable but meaningful stepping stones to success. Begin with what you can do and the rest will follow...

- *Learn to recognise the monkey!* Know the difference between what you're able to address fairly sensibly and what you tend to talk yourself out of, or into, and where, when and with who that happens.

- *Make yourself mindful* - If you choose to indulge make it a *conscious choice*, make it *socially and / or emotionally valuable,* and *give it a time frame.*

- *Befriend instead of berate*: Once a sense of failure no longer serves any purpose, use and develop the most valuable psychological muscle you have: *Let go and move on!*

- *Find alternatives* You don't have to react to everything by eating.

- *Find distractions* to take you through high risk times.

- *Have distractions at the ready!* You've already given them thought so they're at the ready, already!

- *Find whatever lights your fire!!* It fills the gap more than food!

* * *

Whilst a healthy weight and weight maintenance is a matter of eating less, eating differently, and / or moving around more, the sum total of lifestyle, emotional and physical wellbeing create the knock on effect. It is always a chain reaction, and each of you will have your own areas to work on, which are unique to *you*. The combination of factors specific to you alone is what creates your Eating Behaviour Blueprint.

Further, what seems easy for one person, is not for another. Discovering what for *you* is easy, and what is by contrast a work in progress, really does put you ahead of the game. It puts you back in charge, with the only prerequisite being your motivation to continue, and your willingness to plan.

Lastly, it can be difficult not to compare ourselves with others who seem to fare better at mastering their cravings and managing their weight: what you *cannot* always know is how long a person has struggled before an apparent transformation took place, so beware of doing yourself down on the basis of assumption.

The tipping point for transformation might be your mindset, your life situation, the food you eat and your emotional resilience. That magic matrix in motion. Mostly though it comes from recognizing the impact of eating behaviours on your all round health, and knowing that you want a different relationship with food. The tipping point, for lasting change, will always come when something within you has crossed a point of no return. That settled decision. The rest follows.

Appendix

As throughout the book, references are listed as footnotes within the context of each chapter, I have chosen to repeat only those which may provide relevant further reading.

Habit – The Automatic Impulse and Unconscious Behaviour

"The Psychology of Addiction" by Mary McMurran. Taylor & Francis 1994

"Mindfulness: A practical guide to finding peace in a frantic world" by Prof Mark Williams & Dr Danny Penman. PIATKUS – May 2011

Life, Stuff, and the Social Spectrum

"The Genetics of Obesity in Adult Adoptees and their Biological Siblings": T.I. Sorensen, R.A. Price, A.J. Stunkard and F. Schulsinger. BMJ 14/01/1982

"The Genetics of Obesity": T.I. Sorensen Sept 1995

"Facts about Obesity": National Centre for Eating Disorders

"Role of Set Point Theory in Regulation of Weight": R.B.Harris 1990

"Neural Correlates of Food Addiction": Ashley N. Gearhardt et al.

"Jama Psychiatry" – formerly Archives of General Psychiatry Volume 68 No 8 August 2011

"The Yale Food Addiction Scale": Gearhardt, Corbin & Brownell
www.midss.org/content/yale-food-addiction-scale-yfas

Life Cycles and Transitions

"Death: The Final Stage of Growth by" Elisabeth Kubler-Ross. Simon & Schuster Nov 2009

Reactive Eating and the Emotional Spectrum – What lies beneath?

"Living with Death and Dying" by Elisabeth Kubler-Ross. 1997 Scribener

"Working it Through: An Elisabeth Kubler-Ross Workshop on Life, Death and Transitions" - Simon & Schulster 1981

"The 15 Minute Rule" by Caroline Buchanan – Right Way 2012

"Waking the Tiger: Healing Trauma" by Peter Levine. North Atlantic Books 1997

"The Six Pillars of Self Esteem" by Nathaniel Branden. Bantam Books 1995

"The Body Remembers" by Babette Rothschild. W W Norton & Co 11/2011

The Physically Driven Spectrum

Television programme: Horizon 2011/2012 "The Truth about Exercise."

Television programme: Horizon 2012/ 2013 "Eat, Fast, Live Longer."

"FastExercise: the simple secret of high intensity training" by Michael Mosley with Peta Bee. First Atria Books 2014

Lighting Your Fire and Other Distractions

"Sacred Contracts: Awakening your Divine Potential" by Caroline Myss. Bantam Books 2001 *www.myss.com*

"Honouring the Self: Self-Esteem and Personal Transformation" by Nathaniel Branden. Bantam Books 1983 *www.nathanielbranden.com*

How We See Things and Other Beliefs and Assumptions

"Games People Play: The Psychology of Human Relationships" by Eric Berne. Penguin Group 1964 *www.ericberne.com/transactional-analysis*

"Constructing New Core Beliefs: A CBT Master Class (UK)" by Christina Padesky 2013 *www.padesky.com*

On Self Esteem by Nathaniel Branden *www.nathanielbranden.com/on-selfesteem*

"I've Blown It!" and Other Things We Tell Ourselves

"Confidence Works: Learn to be your own Life Coach" by Gladeana McMahon. SPCK Publishing 2001

Managing Situations and How To Say "No."

"Nice Ways to say "No" to Food Pushers" by Erin Whitehead *http://www.sparkpeople.com/resource/nutrition*

"The Drama Triangle" by Stephen Karpman *www.karpmandramatriangle.com*

Working the System

"The Alternate Day Diet": James B Johnson MD & Donald R Laub Sr MD. Michael Joseph / Penguin Books 2008

"The Fast Diet: The Secret of Intermittent Fasting" by Michael Mosley & Mimi Spencer / thefastdiet.co.uk

Tricks of the Trade: Food Wisdom and curbing the urge

"Wheat Belly" by William Davis. Rodale Books 12/2011
"Wheat Belly Cookbook" by William Davis. Rodale Books 01/2014
www.wheatbelly.com

"The X Factor Diet: For Lasting Weight Loss and Vital Health" by Lesley Kenton. Vermilion London 01/2005

"The Carbohydrate Addict's Diet: The Lifelong Solution to Yo Yo Dieting" by Dr Rachael F Fuller & Dr Richard F Fuller. Vermilion London 06/2000

"The South Beach Diet Quick and Easy Cook Book" by Dr Arthur Agatston. Random House 11/2005

"Living Lighter Lite – LighterLife: Life in Balance Recipe Book" www.lighterlife.com

Meals in Minutes – Cambridge Weight Plan www.cambridgeweightplan.com

The 5:2 Diet Book by Kate Harrison. Orion Books Feb 2013

Summing Up

"E-Squared: Nine Do-It-Yourself Energy Experiments That Prove Your Thoughts Create Your Reality" by Pam Grout. Hay House Insights 01/2013

FURTHER READING:

"The 5:2 Diet Book: Feast for 5 days and Fast for just 2 to Lose Weight, Boost your Brain and Transform your Life" by Kate Harrison. Orion Books Feb 2013

"The 5:2 Diet Cookbook: Recipes for the 2 Day Fasting" by Mimi Spencer and Dr Michael Mosley. Rockbridge Press 2013

"The Vice Busting Diet" by Julia Griggs Havey. St Martin's Press 2006

"Eating Less" by Gillian Riley www.eatingless.com/book

"The Chimp Paradox" by Dr Steven Peters 2011 www.chimpparadox.co.uk

"Sweet Poison - why sugar makes us fat" by David Gillespie. Penguin Books 2008

RESOURCES:

National Centre for Eating Disorders *www.eating-disorders.org.uk* *www.eating-disorders.org.uk/counselling/breakthrough-with-deanne-jade/*

Overeaters Anonymous www.oagb.org.uk

MoreLife – *www.more-life.co.uk*
MoreLife deliver weight management and health improvement programmes to individuals, families, local communities and workforces, in addition to operating one of Europe's longest running residential weight management camps for children and young adults.

Khiron House Trauma Clinic *www.khironhouse.com*

www.growthandtransition.com A 3 day residential process led by staff of the EKR centre. Originally more for loved ones and caregivers of the bereaved, but opened up to broader therapeutic transformation after 1985

www.somatictraumatherapy.com the website for Babette Rothschild, a body therapist and specialist educator in the field of trauma and Post Traumatic Stress Disorder

www.recover-from-grief.com/7stages-of-grief

"Byron Katie: The 4 Questions" – The Work of Byron Katie *www.thework.com*

RESOURCES for FEEDING the SOUL!!

Findhorn: *www.findhorn.org/ www.findhorn.com/*

Skyros: *www.skyros.com/*

The Grange: *www.skyros.com/isleofwight*

www.morethanadance.com
Learn or just enjoy Rueda style Cuban Salsa with a great teacher and experienced dance partners so you're rarely on your own.

Acknowledgements

Other than the many, whose stories and valiance of effort have provided so much of my learning, I would like to thank the following more specifically:

Susannah Hughes – for her fantastic friendship and tireless support in so many ways, and "editorial" analysis of the book.

Pamela Bonney – editor in chief and typo flagger extraordinaire, I hope I do her justice!

Christopher Bonney – (website consultant www.thegorillaguide.com) for masterminding this luddite from one computer system to another along with "technical support", in the face of much resistance!

Matt Maguire (www.candescentpress.co.uk) for his patience and perseverance in formatting, and creative transformation of unwieldy diagrams into something light and legible!

Raymond Phillip, for his illustrative contributions.

Christine Bailey – ditto the fantastic friendship and support, an ever fresh perspective, and life enhancing humour!

Martin Harding – principal bank roller during a highly challenging year, without whose "patronage" Overeating Unplugged may well have died!

Finally, Norman Niblock, late proprietor of La Gaillardie, whose wonderful surrounds provided space and time for completion. He is much missed, along with the little hamlet which is a tiny piece of heaven.

About the author

Jill Bonney is an experienced counsellor (B.A.Hons) who has worked with people from all walks of life. For the last 14 years she has specialised in weight loss and weight management, helping hundreds of people to explore their relationship with food, and transform their lives for the better. Her unique insight stems especially from 20 years as airline cabin crew, and coping with her own fatigue-triggered overeating.

Jill lives in London and the Isle of Wight.

www.overeatingunplugged.com

Made in the USA
Coppell, TX
18 August 2022

81694452R00214